Developing Residency Training in Global Health: A Guidebook

iUniverse, Inc.
New York   Bloomington

Contents

Suggested Citation:
Jessica Evert, Chris Stewart, Kevin Chan, Melanie Rosenberg,
Tom Hall, and others. Developing Residency Training in Global
Health: A Guidebook. San Francisco: Global Health Education
Consortium, 2008. 148 pp.

Authors:
Jessica Evert MD, Department of Family and Community Medicine, University of California, San Francisco

Chris Stewart, MD, MA, Assistant Clinical Professor, Department of Pediatrics, University of California at San Francisco

Kevin Chan, MD, MPH, Assistant Professor, The Hospital for Sick Children and Fellow, Munk Centre for International Studies, University of Toronto

Melanie Rosenberg, MD, Pediatric Hospitalist, Children's National Medical Center

Thomas Hall, MD, DrPH, Lecturer, Department of Epidemiology and Biostatistics, University of California at San Francisco

Contributors:
Evaleen Jones MD, President, Child and Family Health International, Associate Professor, Stanford University School of Medicine

Scott Loeliger MS MD, Director, Mark Stinson Fellowship in Underserved and Global Health, Contra Costa Family Practice Residency

Kari Yacisin, Medical Student, Wake Forest University School of Medicine

Regina Crawford Windsor, Master's of Public Health Student, University of Alabama at Birmingham

Laura Warner, Medical Student, Rush Medical College

Acknowledgments:

Thank you for the editing efforts of-

Chris Stewart, MD
Assistant Clinical Professor of Pediatrics
University of California, San Francisco
Director of Global Health Scholars Program

Thuy Bui, MD
Assistant Professor of Medicine
University of Pittsburgh
Global Health Residency Track Director

Flora Teng
Medical Student
University of British Columbia

Thanks to Kathleen Shore DO, Phoenix Baptist Family Medicine, and her team for their energy and efforts in data collection

Thanks to the sponsors of this project: Global Health Education Consortium, American Medical Student Association, Child and Family Health International.

INTRODUCTION

Jessica Evert MD, Department of Family and Community Medicine, University of California, San Francisco

Melanie Rosenberg, MD, Pediatric Hospitalist, Children's National Medical Center

The quest to improve global health represents a challenge of monumental proportions: the problems seem so enormous, the obstacles so great, and success so elusive. On the other hand it is difficult to imagine a pursuit more closely aligned with the professional values and visceral instincts of most physicians. Many young doctors enter medicine with a passionate interest in global health; our challenge is to nurture this commitment and encourage its expression.[1]

Globalization is taking hold of all sectors of society. Not surprisingly, many residency applicants are interested in global health training opportunities during their graduate medical education. Meanwhile, residency programs grapple with the challenges of establishing and expanding global health programming. The past decade has witnessed a rise in number of non-profit organizations dedicated to global health exposure for future physicians. Child and Family Health International, Doctors for Global Health, and Community for Children are a few examples. In addition, interest has increased within specialty societies, leading to the establishment of international subcommittees and seminars, such as the annual International Family Medicine Development Workshop and the International Child Health Section of the American Academy of Pediatrics. The mission of the Global Health Education Consortium is to support and augment these educational activities.

This is an exciting time for global health program development. As with any program introduction or expansion, the challenges are many. This guidebook tries to navigate the maze of global health education, provide examples of global health residency training, and identify resources for developing and improving programs. In the midst of this endeavor, we must keep in mind the founding oath of medical practice. Just as physicians swear to "do no harm" to their patients, we must be mindful of inadvertent harms of global health work and conscientiously try to avoid them.

1.D Shaywitz and D Ausiello. "Global Health: A Chance for Western Physicians to Give and Receive." The American Journal of Medicine. 2002;113(4)354-7.

A PDF version of this document is available at: www.globalhealthedu.org under "Resources".

Chapter 1

Global Health Education: History And Literature Review

Jessica Evert MD, Department of Family and Community Medicine, University of California, San Francisco

Melanie Rosenberg, MD, Pediatric Hospitalist, Children's National Medical Center

A Brief History*

Although the idea that medicine and health transcend geographic boundaries is not new, it is taking a long time for it to be fully integrated into U.S. medical education and practice. Over the last 20 years, globalization of all sectors of society, including business, media and education, has been expedited and facilitated by the internet/computer revolution. However, the discipline of international health (or as it is now being termed, "global health") in its current form has evolved over the last 150 years.

The roots of international health can be traced to the cholera outbreak of the mid-1800s. This disease crisis prompted physicians and politicians to convene the first International Sanitary Conference in 1851. Successive conferences focused on the "germ de jour," such as yellow fever and bubonic plague, for the remainder of the 19th century. These conferences took place annually until 1938, eventually becoming meetings in which the leading discoveries in medicine were presented and served as a vehicle for the development of shared medical diction.

In 1902 hemispheric collaboration to deal with yellow fever led to the creation of the Pan American Sanitary Bureau (now called the Pan American Health Organization), which soon became a model for transnational information sharing and health promotion. Following World War I, organizations from different corners of the globe (the leading one being the League of Nations Health Committee) expanded international health from a focus on infectious disease to a discipline addressing maternal and infant health, nutrition, housing, physical education, drug trafficking, and occupational health.

The brutalities of World War II Nazi concentration camps gave rise to a new degree of humanism that led to unprecedented cooperation as the world vowed to prevent repetition of such suffering. As is evident, many of the early events leading up to modern-day international health were focused on health crises in the Americas and Europe. In 1948, the World Health Organization (WHO) was created out of the UN's desire to have a single global entity charged with fostering cooperation and collaboration among member countries to address health problems. The mission of WHO embodied a new concept of health: it was not merely the absence of disease but the promotion, attainment, and maintenance of physical, mental, and social well-being.

In 1948 the first Student International Clinical Conference brought together medical students throughout Europe. In 1951, this conference evolved into the International Federation of Medical Students' Associations with the stated objective of "studying and promoting the interests of medical student co-operation on a purely professional basis, and promoting activities in the field of student health and student relief." This mission was soon expanded to include medical student cooperation to improving the health of all populations. In 1947, doctors from 27 countries met in Paris and created the World Medical Association, whose objective is "to serve humanity by endeavoring to achieve the highest international standards in Medical Education, Medical Science, Medical Art and Medical Ethics, and Health Care for all people in the world."

WHO's failure to eradicate malaria (after a significant victory over smallpox) revealed the interrelationship of health and infrastructure, culture, politics and economic stability. In addition, it demonstrated the imperative that health campaigns be culturally-sensitive and discredited the notion of magic bullets for the world's disease burdens. Medecins Sans Frontieres (Doctors Without Borders) was created in 1971 by physicians dissatisfied with the inadequate efforts of WHO and the International Red Cross to address structural and political barriers that led to health crises. In 1977, WHO shifted from a disease-specific to a health-for-all approach.

The increasing focus on international health is evident in several large U.S.A. organizations. The International Health Medical Education Consortium (now called the Global Health Education Consortium), created in 1991, now has a membership of approximately 80 medical schools in the U.S.A. and Canada and aims to foster international health education for medical students. The American Medical Association opened its Office of International Medicine in 1978, the U.S.A. chapter of International Federation of Medical Students' Association (IFMSA) was started in 1998 and the Global Health Action Committee of the American Medical Student Association in 1997. Today, many specialty professional organizations have global health subcommittees.

Today, we are increasingly aware that health is determined by interrelated medical, political, economic, educational, and environmental factors. Consequently, the future of world health requires partnerships between nations, health care professionals, medical researchers, public health specialists, corporations, and individuals. Currently, the economic, human, and environmental consequences of the health disparities in the world are being elucidated. For example, in 2001 the WHO Macroeconomic Commission on Health put forth three core findings:

1. The massive amount of disease burden in the world's poorest nations poses a huge threat to global wealth and security.
2. Millions of impoverished people around the world die of preventable and treatable infectious diseases because they lack access to basic medical care and sanitation.
3. We have the ability and technology to save millions of lives each year if only the wealthier nations would help provide poorer countries with such health care and services. [1]

These principles sound simple and straightforward, but their implementation is complex and expensive. We have reached a point in the history of international medicine where trained professional and technical personnel from many fields are cooperating to meet the multifaceted challenges to world health. Each field is training individuals equipped to participate in these efforts. Just as medicine is training doctors who specialize in international health, law is training lawyers who specialize in international law. Medical educators around the world are trying to identify skills sets necessary for collaboration and to find ways to cultivate them among interested trainees.

Literature Review of Global Health Graduate Medical Education

Background.-- An article in the November 1969 issue of the Journal of the American Medical Association reported, "every U.S.A. medical school is involved in such international activities as faculty travel for study, research and teaching, clinical training for foreign graduates, and medical student study overseas...a recent self-survey by Case Western Reserve medical students indicated that 78% of the first-year class and 85% of the second-year class were interested in studying or working abroad at sometime in their medical school careers."[2] The article went on to report that 600 American medical students went abroad during the academic year 1966-1967. This interest in global health continues today. Results of recent surveys by the Association of American Medical Colleges show that the proportion of American medical students taking an international elective during medical school has increased significantly over the last decade, from under 15% in 1998 to almost 30% in 2006.[3] More and more medical schools have begun offering formal training in global health. As this training increases, so will the demand for continued and more specialized training during residency.

Effects of International Electives on Students and Residents: Public Health Knowledge, Clinical Skills, and Cultural Sensitivity.-- Efforts have been made to investigate the benefits of such international electives on medical students and residents. One study showed that medical students who participated in a 3-6-week international program scored significantly higher in the preventive medicine/public health sections of the USMLE board exam than a control group.[4] In another study, medical student participants said their international experience sharpened awareness of the importance of public health and patient education.[5] Seventy-eight percent of the students also reported a heightened awareness of cost issues and financial barriers to patient care. All students in this group also reported that they appreciated the utility of a history and physical examination over the use of diagnostic tests. In a study of medical students and residents who participated in international health electives, attitudes toward the importance of doctor-patient communication, use of symbolism by patients, public health interventions, and community health programs were more positive after than before their experience. When participants were re-interviewed 2 years later, they reported continued positive influences from the experience on their clinical and language skills, sensitivity to cultural and socioeconomic factors, awareness of the role of communication in clinical care, and attitudes toward careers working with the underserved (p<.01).[6] A similar positive impact on self-assessed cultural competence and sense of idealism was found in a study of clinical medical students who had completed an international elective.[7] In comparison with students who did not choose an international elective, students in their third year of medical school showed significantly higher levels of idealism, enthusiasm, and interest in primary care, as well as sharpened perception of the need to understand cultural differences. Similar effects have been found in medical residents receiving international health training or completing an elective. Participants in an international health program in internal medicine were more likely than non-participants to believe that U.S. physicians underused their physical exam and history-taking skills and reported that the experience had a positive influence on their clinical diagnostic skills.[8] An internal medicine elective program was found to have a positive impact on tropical medicine knowledge for participants,[9] and participants in a pediatric international health elective reported seeing a significant number of diseases and clinical presentations that they had never encountered at their home institution.[10] Notably missing from the current literature is an evaluation of the impacts residents have on their international hosts.

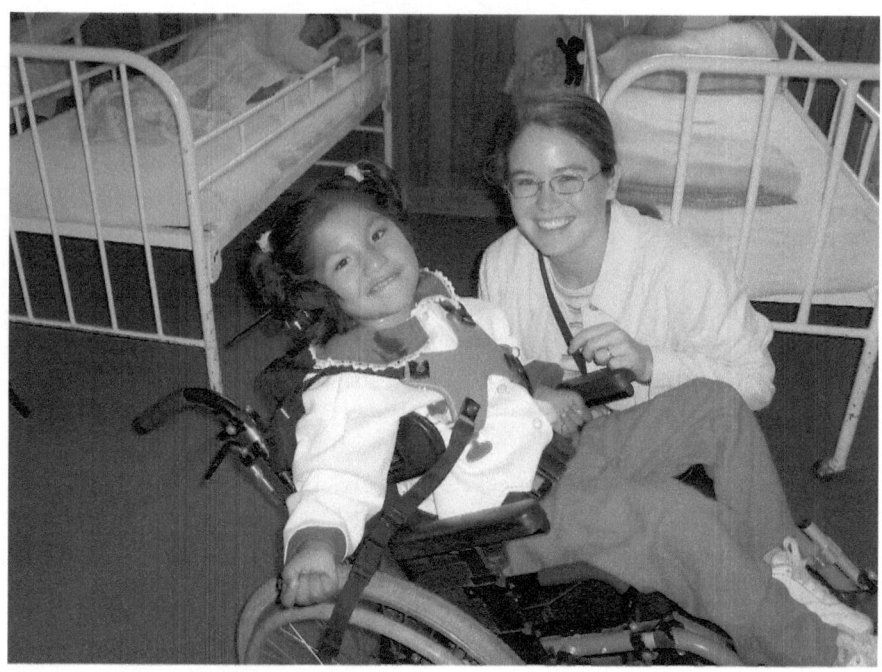

Lawrence Family Medicine resident Abby Rattin, MD in Peru.

Impact on Career Choice-- Studies have also shown that international health experience during training may influence career choice. Medical students who participated in an international health experience in a developing country were more likely later to practice in underserved areas in the U.S.A.[11]   During 1995-1997, 60 senior medical students were chosen to participate in the International Health Fellowship, an intensive 2-week course followed by about 2 months in a developing country. When participants were surveyed several years after completing the fellowship, most of them reported it had significantly influenced their careers. The majority were practicing primary care, and over half had participated in community health projects or had done further work overseas.[12]   Internal medicine residents who participated in international electives were found more likely to change career plans from subspecialty to general medicine[8] and toward general medicine or public health.[9] An association between international health experience and practicing primary care, public health, or working in underserved communities seems consistent across studies. Although this may be due to selection bias, it may also reflect an important outcome of global health exposure on career choice.

Effect on Ranking of Residency Programs-- The demand for training and experience in international health is evident from studies examining the role international health opportunities play in applicants' ranking of residency programs. At a pediatric residency program in Colorado where a formal International Health Elective is offered, 67% of residents cited the opportunity as a major factor in ranking the program.[10] Similarly, 42% of residents surveyed at Duke University's Internal Medicine Residency Program cited their well-established International Health Program as a significant factor in ranking.[9] In 1993, at the University of Cincinnati Family Medicine Residency Program, an official International Health Track was implemented through which residents were able to complete an international elective and receive year-round didactic training. The creators noted that since the 1990s the pool of U.S.A.-graduated medical students applying to family medicine programs had been declining and recruiting had become more competitive. A survey of all program graduates from 1994 to 2003 found that participants in the International Health track ranked it as the most important factor in choosing the program. Residents in the track were more likely to have relocated farther from both their medical school and home city for residency than non-participants, indicating the appeal of the track. Simultaneously, during the years following implementation of this program, match rates for the program improved from 70% to 100%, again supporting the notion that international health opportunities are important in recruiting residents.[13] Since these studies were done at programs offering international health opportunities, the results cannot be generalized to the entire applicant pool. No studies have been done of all applicants in any one field to determine the overall importance of international health in residency ranking. However, a survey of all first-year Emergency Medicine residents (2000-2001) in the United States found that 62% of respondents who had interviewed at programs with international opportunities considered this a positive factor in the ranking process, 58% perceived the need for additional training in an international setting, and 76% indicated that would like more international EM exposure in their current residency program.[4]

Availability of Global Health Training--Most specialties have gathered, or are in the process of gathering, data on the availability of international training in their disciplines. Within family medicine, a 1998 survey found that 54% of programs offered global health training and 15% offered curricular and financial support for it. Logistic regression analysis of these data suggested that the longevity of the global health programming, covering of living expenses at the international site, and involvement of faculty in international work in the past two years were correlated with increased likelihood of participation of residents in global health activities.[15] A 2007 survey of U.S.A. surgical residents found that 98% were interested in international electives even though global health electives and programs are limited within surgical programs.[16] Although no surveys have been published in the realm of orthopedic surgery, the University of California, San Francisco, orthopedic surgery residency reports 41% its residents took part in international electives, prompting it to establish a longitudinal program with Orthopedics Overseas in Umtata, South Africa.[17] International Emergency Medicine Fellowships have also been created, with the following stated goals : (1) To develop the ability to assess international health systems and identify pertinent emergency health issues; (2) To design emergency health programs that address identified needs; (3) To develop the skills necessary to implement emergency programs abroad and integrate them into existing health systems; and (4) To develop the ability to evaluate the quality and effectiveness of international health programs.[18] A 1995 survey of pediatric programs found that 25% of respondents offered international electives, although most programs did not report having a formal education structure.[19] A recent cross-sectional survey of all pediatric residency programs accredited by the Accreditation Council for Graduate Medical Education (ACGME) revealed a substantial increase in availability of global health electives.[20] Of the programs that responded (53%), over half had offered a global health elective in the preceding year, and 47% had incorporated global health education into their residency curricula. Programs reported providing support to residents in various ways, including faculty mentorship, clinical training and orientation, post-elective debriefing, and funding. Currently, there is a paucity of studies comparing the quality and content of global health programming within and between disciplines.

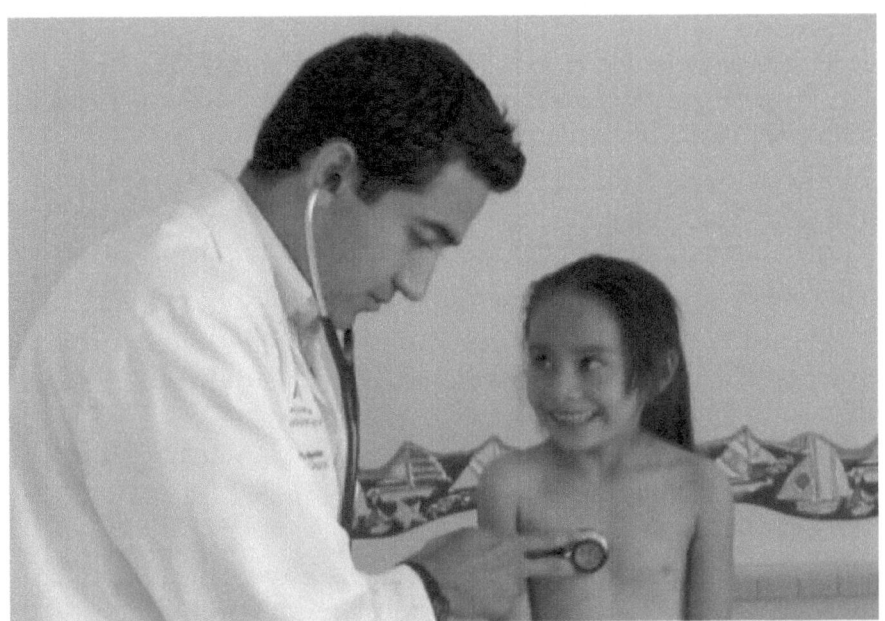

Rainbow Babies and Children's Hospital International Health Track participant David Naimi, MD working in a pediatric clinic in Oaxaca, Mexico.

Barriers to Training: Establishing residency programs in global health encounter numerous hurdles, and, as for most other types of program expansion, the main one is financial. One issue is the varying interpretation of the Center for Medicare and Medicaid Services rules on graduate medical education payments for residents rotating abroad. Another constraint is the curricular requirements set by ACGME and specialty boards. Program and partnership sustainability is another hurdle to quality programming, particularly when international partnerships demand ethical considerations of the long-term effects on local communities, patients, and health-care practitioners.[21] One survey of surgical residents showed the most significant barriers were financial difficulties and scheduling (82% and 52%).[16] Difficulties in creating and sustaining international partnerships, establishing and maintaining institutional support, and evaluating programs effectively are also encountered.

    * Heavily borrowed from Developing Global Health Curricula: A Guidebook for U.S.A. and Canadian Medical Schools.

References

1. *Macroeconomics and Health: Investing in Health for Economic Development: Report of the Commission on Macroeconomics and Health.* Jeffrey D. Sachs, Chair. Presented 20 December 2001.

2. International Medical Education. JAMA 1969;210(8):1555-57.

3. Association of American Medical Colleges. 2006 Medical School Graduate Questionnaire. Available at www.aamc.org/data/gq/ allschoolreports/2006.pdf. Accessed April 5, 2007.

4. Waddell WH, Kelley PR, Suter E, Levit EJ. Effectiveness of an international health elective as measured by NBME Part II. J Med Educ. 1976 Jun;51(6):468-72.

5. Bissonette R, Route C. "The Educational Effect of Clinical Rotations in Nonindustrialized Countries." Family Medicine 1994;26:226-31.

6. Haq C, Rothenberg D, Gjerde C, et al. "New world views: preparing physicians in training for global health work." Family Medicine 2000;32:566-72.

7. Godkin MA, Savageau JA. "The Effect of a Global Multiculturalism Track on Cultural Competence of Preclinical Medical Students." Family Medicine. 2001;33(3):178-86.

8. Gupta et al. "The International Health Program: The Fifteen-Year Experience With Yale University's Internal Medicine Residency Program." American Journal of Tropical Medicine and Hygiene 1999;61(6):1019-1023.

9. Miller WC, Corey GR, Lallinger GJ, Durack DT. International Health and internal medicine residency training: the Duke University experience. Am J Med 1995;99(3):291-7.

10. Federico, et al. A Successful International Child Health Elective: The University of Colorado's Department of Pediatrics experience. Arch Pediatr Adolesc Med. 2006 Feb;160(2):191-6.

11. Chiller TM, De Mieri P, Cohen I. "International Health Training. The Tulane Experience." Infectious Disease Clinics of North America. 1995;9:439-43.

12. Ramsey AH, Haq C, Gjerde CL, Rothenberg D. Career influence of an international health experience during medical school. Fam Med. 2004 Jun;36(6):412-6.

13. Bazemore AW, Henein M, Goldenhar LM, Szaflarski M, Lindsell CJ, Diller P. The Effect of Offering International Health Training Opportunities on Family Medicine Residency Recruiting. Fam Med. 2007; 39(4):255-60.

14. Dey CC, Grabowski JG, Gebreyes, et al. Influence of International Emergency Medicine opportunities on Residency Program Selection. Acad Emerg Med. 2002; 9 (7):679-683

15. Schultz SH, Rousseau S. International health training in family practice residency programs. Family Medicine. 1998 Jan; 30(1):29-33.

16. Powell AC, Mueller C, Kingham P, International experience, electives, and volunteerism in surgical training: a survey of resident interest. J Am Coll Surg. 2007 Jul; 205(1):162-8.

17. Haskell A, Rovinsky D, Brown HK, Coughlin RR. The UCSF international orthopaedic elective. Clin Orthop. 2002 Mar; 396:12-18.

18. Anderson PD, Aschkenasy M, Lis J. International emergency medicine fellowships. Emerg Med Clin North Am. 2005 Feb; 23(1):199-215.

19. Torjesen K, Mandalakas A, Kahn R, Duncan B. International child health electives for pediatric residents. Arch Pediatr Adolesc Med. 1999 Dec;153(12):1297-302.

20. Nelson BD, Lee ACC, Newby PK, Chamberlin MR, Huang C. Global health training in pediatric residency programs. Pediatrics. July, 2008; 122 (1):28-33

21. Evert J, Bazemore A, Hixon A, Withy K. Going global: considerations for introducing global health into family medicine training programs. Fam Med. 2007 Oct;39(9):659-65.

Chapter 2

Types Of Global Health Programming

Christopher C. Stewart, MD, MA, Assistant Clinical Professor, Department of Pediatrics, University of California at San Francisco

Lisa Dillabaugh, MD, Resident, Department of Pediatrics, University of California at San Francisco

Kevin Chan, MD, MPH, Assistant Professor, The Hospital for Sick Children, and Fellow, Munk Centre for International Studies, University of Toronto

As interest in global health has increased among both medical students and residents, residency programs are challenged with providing trainees with opportunities to expand their knowledge and pursue experiences in this emerging field. Most major medical schools are developing global health programs, largely on the basis of resident demand. Admissions and program directors are increasingly aware that residents consider global health opportunities in their selection process. Given this interest among applicants, global health residencies will play a key role as residency programs try to attract high-quality trainees.

The vision for a medical school's residency program in global health can range from establishing overseas rotations to developing didactic experiences, and even incorporating Master's degrees or fellowships into the curriculum. Many global health programs simply involve rotations at one or more international sites. At the other end of the spectrum, a wide variety of programs offer varied curriculum in both international and local global health-related experiences. Some of these have been around for decades; many more are being established in response to increasing resident demand. Chapter 5 describes various programs in depth to see how their components might be combined to create a residency global health program or track that makes sense for a particular medical school.

Time is a critical factor in providing comprehensive global health education during residency. Medical school offers much more opportunity for elective courses and longitudinal experiences, particularly in the first two years. Time in residency is restricted by Residency Review Committee (RRC) and ACGME requirements, which can affect elective time. Work hour restrictions might make evening sessions difficult and even impossible to require. Programs must be creative to provide opportunities for undertaking projects, doing research, or even spending large amounts of time abroad. The time factor has led some programs to consider adding an extra year to residency that could be directed in part to earning a Master's or other graduate degree.

Global health education isn't valuable only for those with strong interests in global health careers. Trainees who participate in international electives improve their physical exam skills, become more cost conscious, and show greater commitment to underserved populations. Thus, the resident audience for global health education spans those without any identified interest in international health to those anticipating careers in it. Providing global health education to residents comes in many forms, some of which are outlined below.

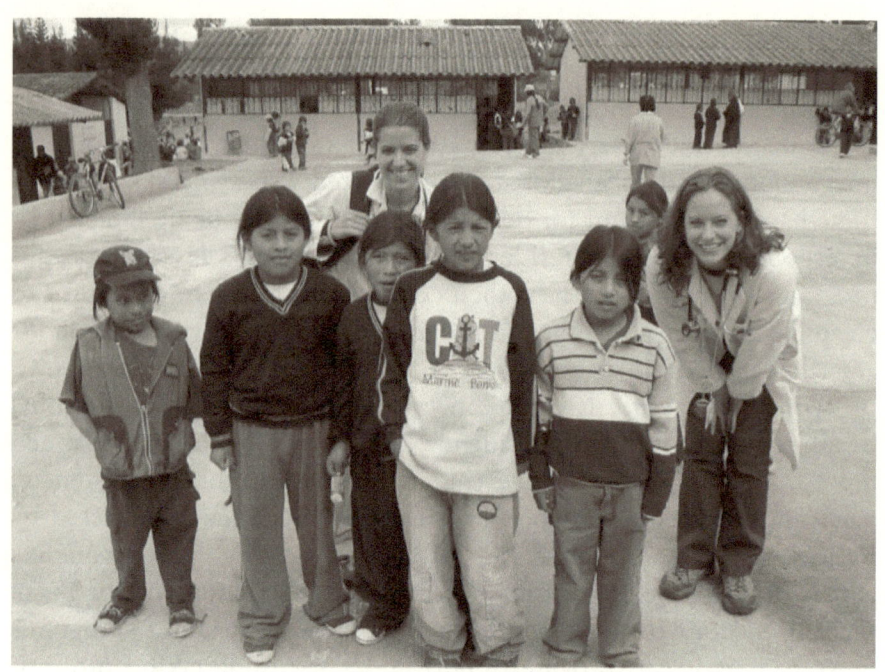

Rainbow Babies and Children's Hospital International Health Track
participants Leah Millstein, MD and Allison Ross, MD in Ecuador with
InterHealth South America.

Curricular Content

For more comprehensive programs, it would make sense to write out goals, objectives, and even a mission statement. These can be guides as a program develops. Some examples of these are found in the detailed program descriptions in Chapter 4.

One basic objective for a global health residency might be to meet residents' demand for structured and supervised experiential learning opportunities abroad. These should include proper supervision, clear goals, pre-trip preparation and post-trip debriefing, evaluation from both supervisors abroad and residents themselves, and some type of report or dissemination of the experience. Resources for these can be found in Chapter 8. Objectives of a more comprehensive global health program might include the following:

• To provide coursework and other educational options for concentrated learning within the discipline of global health;

- To provide mentorship in research, program development and evaluation, and education program development in resource-poor countries; and

- To expose residents to research, academic, and other career opportunities in global health.

What Constitutes a Global Health Curriculum?

The idea of developing core competencies in global health has come up as the global health education field is challenged to define itself. Core competencies might exist within specialties or for the field as a whole and might vary with field of residency. Surgeons and psychiatrists, for example, might view the focus of global health training quite differently. An example of core competencies for pediatrics in global health being developed by the American Academy of Pediatrics can be found in Chapter 7.

On a more general note, a variety of questions come up: How does global health relate to public health? Are epidemiology and biostatistics part of the global health core skill set? Is global health just public health in new clothes? What degree of political understanding, economic training, ethics, etc. is needed to prepare those who wish to pursue careers in global health? These are challenging questions for those in medical education trying to develop a global health curriculum. Some answers can be seen in the examples featured in Chapter 4.

For residents, development of excellent clinical skills and broad training in their specialty are central to their programs and should not be sacrificed for peripheral training. However, skills in leadership, program management, and program evaluation are important to the types of jobs often done by those in global health careers and may therefore need to be offered.

General content areas for a global health curriculum would include the following: an overview of global health and the global burden of disease; health indicators and an understanding of their use and limitations; economic and social development; institutions and organizations involved in global health, including policy and trade agreements; environmental health, including water issues, natural and man-made disasters, and immigration issues; zoonoses; cultural, social and behavioral determinants of health; demography; social justice and global health including an understanding of human rights; staying healthy during the global health field experience; global health ethics and professionalism, and cultural competency training. Core content might also include specific diseases or topics such as malaria, tuberculosis, HIV, measles, nutrition, and maternal and child health, considered separately or woven into other subjects.

Laboratory skills might also be taught, with a review of gram stains, malaria preps, and other procedures often referred to specialists or technicians in affluent countries. Basic radiology competence, even physical exam skills, might be included, as many residents feel the lack of these in situations where they have no access to the resources they are used to.

Resources for including the above topics into a global health curriculum are reviewed in Chapter 8, and examples of such curriculum in the form of programs are offered in Chapter 4. See Chapter 5 for further discussion of curriculum development and evaluation.

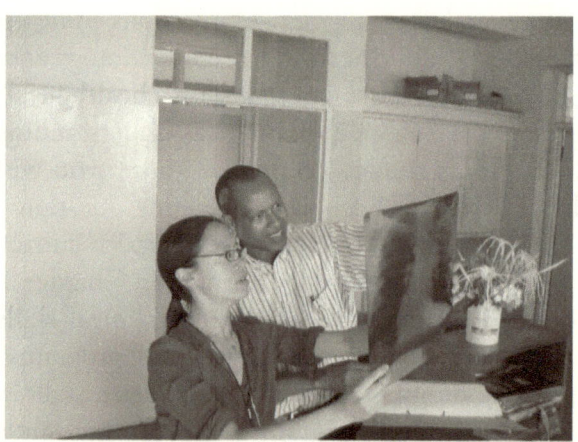

Photo by Guy Vanderberg

UCSF Global Health Clinical Scholars Program planning committee member and graduate of UCSF Internal Medicine Residency Sophy Wong and Dr. Elitumaini Mziray discussing a chest x-ray at Karatu District Hospital in Karatu, Tanzania.

Didactics

While the transition from medical school to residency changes the focus of medical education from lecture-based learning to primarily clinical training, didactic formats still provide a strong base for learning core information. Lectures with a global health focus can be integrated into regular resident conferences and grand rounds. Similarly, journal clubs reviewing historically important, current, or controversial global health topics provide valuable opportunities for residents to gain knowledge. Many institutions also have global health interest groups that hold evening lectures, providing residents with both didactic material and the opportunity to network with faculty and community practitioners working in global health.

On-line modules for teaching topics are becoming more popular. Some examples are presented in Chapter 8. Video-taped lectures are now available, and likely will increase in number with the application of technology to medical education. Ensuring that residents absorb the material they are given can be more challenging, although some of the on-line material comes with quizzes or pre- and post-tests that instructors can use.

Another didactic teaching model takes advantage of the rotation-based structure used by most residency programs to devote up to a month to global health in lieu of an elective rotation. This affords committed residents the time to dedicate their energy to learning about global health, develop projects or research, and plan their careers. As mentioned, some programs offer an expanded residency option in global health with an extra year, which allows didactic time to be incorporated in a more concentrated format.

International Experiences

Many residency programs support travel to developing countries for short periods during training. This often takes the form of a month-long visit to an established site with which the resident's home institution has formed a collaborative relationship. Some of the strongest formalized international health electives identify mentors abroad and at home, prepare residents with pre-departure orientation, and make every effort to find ways for visiting residents to contribute meaningfully to the host institution or organization.

Trainees with particular interests and ingenuity also pursue electives independently through various means, including working with faculty mentors with overseas connections, contacting universities and hospitals directly, or getting involved with non-governmental organizations. Although these electives allow residents to tailor experiences to their interests, they can be complicated by uncertain mentorship and supervision abroad. Some programs allow residents to take leaves of absence from training or are flexible enough for residents to take several months or more off for international health research or projects. Projects of this magnitude often require residents to obtain funding and direct their projects themselves. Other issues related to funding for resident international experiences are covered in Chapter 5.

Exchanges

If the goals or mission statement of a global health program include helping improve conditions for international partners, mutual exchanges should be considered. Many global health programs focus exclusively on residents' travel to other countries and do little to support travel in the other direction. True exchange programs should have true exchange. Although visiting residents or doctors from less developed countries may be restricted in offering patient care, they still have open to them many beneficial opportunities for education, observation, and participation in activities. Some examples are described in Chapter 4. One obvious issue is funding; however, anytime funds are procured for residents to go abroad to a "partner" site, those funds might also be used to bring that site's residents or faculty in the other direction. Although some might argue that the money to pay for resident travel helps partner sites, there are counter-arguments. Short trips often accomplish little for host countries unless they are part of a longitudinal, well-planned, and properly supervised program. Visiting residents can contribute to the "brain drain" of a resource-poor country's institutions by taking up skilled personnel's time for orientation and teaching. Any program visited by international residents or faculty is made keenly aware of the resources and time it takes to host them. True, mutually beneficial exchange programs are difficult and costly, but if a program is going to fulfill its goals of helping resource-scarce country partners, some reasonable exchanges should form part of the equation.

Mentoring

Mentorship is an essential part of all resident training and is no less important for those interested in global health. Residency programs can facilitate it by identifying and supporting faculty members who participate in global health work and research or have substantial experience in developing countries. A mentor for a particular resident does not necessarily need to be limited to one department (Medicine for example), as residents can benefit from cross-disciplinary interactions and can thus determine the best fit for their mentor, based on topics or locations of mutual interest. Valuable mentors can also be found in resource-scarce countries that residents visit during international electives. Mentorship agreements should be in writing and meeting times set to review progress.

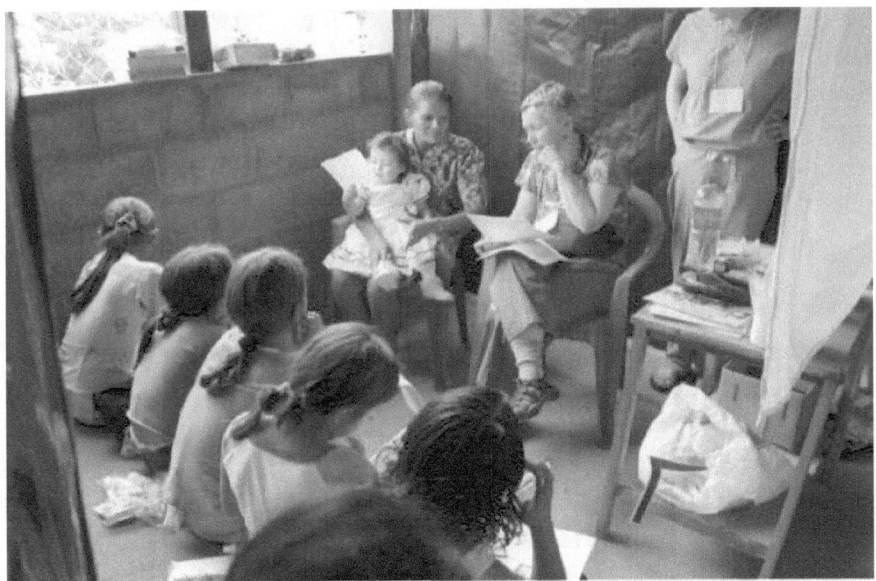

Photo by Kate Nielsen

University of Washington faculty mentor Dr. Elinor Graham presents Charlas topics with residents and community health workers.

Research

Residents can also learn about global health through collaborative research with institutions in developing countries. Residents may work with investigators conducting research overseas, giving them the chance to learn about basic science and clinical research methods, specific global health topics, and research ethics. Time is often a limiting factor for residents: if a resident intends to do research, expectations must be reasonable to allow for a successful outcome. More often than not, it is easier for a resident to do part of an established project themselves, under the supervision of a faculty research mentor. Those who work in international research know only too well that projects move much more slowly than one anticipates. Just getting Institutional Review Board or the Committee on Human Research approval at international sites can take months, even years. Research ethics must be considered: who benefits from research, what is done with the results, and authorship of publications all become important issues in international collaboration. Ideally, these issues are tackled directly up front to avoid misunderstandings and resentments as projects move forward. Further discussion of international research can be found in Chapters 3 and 5.

Domestic Educational Experiences in Global Health

Over the last decade, international health has morphed into the term "global health" as a result of increased globalization coupled with the realization that many health concerns are not limited to poor countries but shared by all. Although on the international level the global health movement focuses on low- and middle-income countries, in general it is concerned with underserved and underprivileged people no matter where they live. Local populations in any country or community struggle with issues of health disparity, providing residency programs with local opportunities to expose resident physicians to global health concerns. Opportunities abound: homeless shelters, refugee or immigrant health clinics, travel clinics, and tuberculosis and HIV clinics, to name a few. Visits to patients living in rooming houses or subsidized housing can be powerful experiences. Collaboration with immigrant advocacy groups, legal assistance programs, and similar agencies can help residents acquire skills in working with diverse

20

communities, leadership skills, and awareness of issues in communities and neighborhoods they served. Language is another key issue. People whose first language is neither English, Spanish, nor French and whose socio-cultural background is different face barriers to care and opportunity.

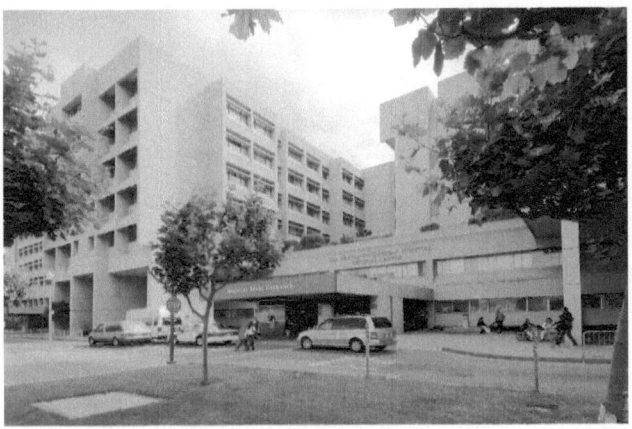

San Francisco General Hospital, home of the Refugee Health Clinic, where UCSF Family Medicine residents receive training in care for refugee and asylee populations.

Global Health Conferences

Residents should be encouraged to attend and present their research or projects at international and national global health conferences. These usually offer excellent didactic teaching and a variety of networking and career opportunities. Examples of such conferences are found in Chapter 8.

Other Experiences

Some experiential learning might be gained through simulation exercises, such as weekend or overnight experiences that mimic responses to complex humanitarian emergencies. Such experiences might teach team building and leadership skills by taking part in real-life scenarios.

Complementary Degree Programs and Fellowships

Many residents enter training after obtaining additional professional degrees or with an interest in doing so. Those interested in global health tend to pursue a Master's in Public Health (MPH), but there are other options, such as master's degrees in economics, public policy, and business administration. Some institutions offer degree programs with a focus on global health or have an area of concentration within the program dedicated to it. Master and doctoral degrees in global health are possibilities at some institutions. These complementary degree programs provide residents with knowledge and skills beyond clinical medicine, although earning them may require taking time off from training, incorporating degrees into research years or fellowship training, or waiting until after residency. As noted above, some medical schools are beginning to offer residency tracks with an extra year, providing an MPH/residency combination, as well as substantial time abroad to work on projects or research. Examples of these can be found in Chapter 4.

Fellowships in global health are becoming more available, although funding is often a barrier. Some programs offer international opportunities in their traditional specialty fellowships; others have specific global health fellowships. These are better than short rotations to international partner sites, which might offer little to the partner and drain scarce resources by taking up their host's time. Fellowships allow for extended time abroad and greater chances for true collaboration and benefits for the partner/host country.

Residents often ask about the potential costs and benefits of additional academic training in global health, e.g., earning an MPH degree. Are such degrees helpful? The answer is: "It depends." It depends on the career the resident wants to pursue. For those engaged in short-term global health assignments or working primarily as clinicians, a public health degree adds little and costs a year of time and money. However, a public health degree can be valuable for substantial global health assignments and a wide variety of jobs concerned with field research and overseas training, especially in jobs concerned with program development, implementation, and evaluation,. The field of concentration will have some bearing on your employability, but probably not as much as the mere possession of a public health degree.

This degree is evidence that you have had basic training in such core disciplines as epidemiology, biostatistics, program planning and management, along with one or more of content areas such as maternal and child health, health education, and environmental health.

In planning a program involving complementary degrees and further certification, residents need to know what is available at their home institution or nearby facilities, available funding, and the potential benefit to the residents' career development. Answering these basic questions may illuminate the need for complementary degrees and certificates.

As this chapter has shown, residents have many avenues open to them in creating a global health program. They could start with a needs assessment of their institution's faculty and residents. Chapter 4 describes examples of successful global health residency programs, whose directors could be contacted for information. Chapter 8 lists resources for global health curriculum.

Chapter 3

Ethics For Global Health Programming

Evaleen Jones MD, President, Child and Family Health International
Associate Professor, Stanford University School of Medicine

Scott Loeliger MS MD, Director, Mark Stinson Fellowship in
Underserved and Global Health, Contra Costa Family Practice
Residency

An Historical Perspective of Medical Ethics
Primum no nocerum~ Above all, Do No Harm...

Above all, Do No Harm --For physicians, this is a hallowed expression of hope and humility, offering recognition that human acts with good intentions may have unwanted consequences. It remains the mantra that guides decisions and treatment from a medical viewpoint, reminding us that we must consider the harm that any intervention might do. Outside the protected environment of the medical campus, however, little has been written about what harm might occur when residents work abroad. Helping out at a hospital or clinic in Tanzania, delivering babies in the bush, working within a PEPFAR-funded AIDS center, weighing infants in feeding centers, or simply attending a community meeting organized by village health workers-- all will require us to consider how the resident's presence and actions affects individuals, communities and health systems.

Several historical documents central to the ethos of Medicine provide us with important guiding principles. Residents preparing to go overseas should review them to gain a deeper, more personal understanding of how these concepts can be applied to physicians practicing abroad. Such ideals are humbling, inviting, inclusive and inspirational...and create the necessary framework and motivation for promoting change.

Declaration of Geneva or The Physician's Oath (Geneva, September 1948)
The Universal Declaration of Human Rights (Geneva, December 1948)
The European Convention on Human Right, (Rome, 1950);
The Declaration of Alma-Ata; Report of the International Conference on
Primary Health Care, September 1978 (WHO Publication, 1978)

Perhaps the document most relevant to global health is the *Declaration of Alma-Ata,* which established ethical boundaries for North American and European physicians. Its primary statement "strongly reaffirms that health, which is a state of complete physical, mental and social wellbeing, and not **merely** the absence of disease and infirmity, is a fundamental **human right** and that the attainment of the highest possible level of health is a most important **world-wide social goal** whose realization requires the action of many other social and economic sectors in addition to the health sector."[1]

Lessons Learned from Global Volunteers

What is the harm in helping? How can we be sure we know what is needed?

One of the early models of overseas service by American college graduates was the highly publicized Peace Corps. It derived from a time when the U.S.A. was looking abroad at its non-military responsibilities. During the presidency of John F. Kennedy, the Peace Corps, its ideals articulated and its mission promoted by Sargent Shriver, encouraged young Americans to go abroad to help those less fortunate.

The Peace Corps' motto of the 1960s and 1970s, "The Hardest Job You Will Ever Love," was quite clear about who benefits from a two-year stint abroad: it was taken as fact that the mere presence of a college graduate would automatically make life better for people in foreign lands. Most returned Peace Corps volunteers, including one of the authors of this chapter, later reflected that it was really us who benefited the most. The true impact of these efforts was less clear and there was even some suspicion that some harm might have come from "doing good." Recently, the community of returned Peace Corps volunteers – a group numbering about 190,000 – has been debating the appropriateness of an expanded Peace Corps sending new graduates to global jobs that they are poorly prepared for or trained to do.[2,3] Such debate is pertinent for those promoting a large scale transfer of medical manpower to the corners of the world.

The exponential increase in global health funding over the last decade has provoked questions about how we help, asking whether our efforts to export expertise, money, and health care largesse are not only often ineffective but at times both wrong-headed and counter-productive.[4,5] How can we be certain that residents serving abroad will not cause distraction and detriment?

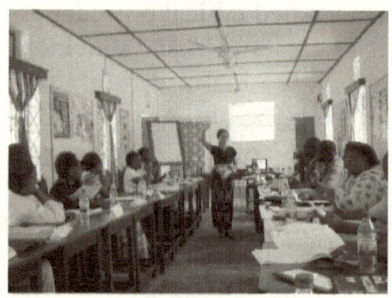

Photo by Royce Lin

Former UCSF Internal Medicine resident Sophy Wong, MD teaching a course on TB-HIV co-infection at Kitete Hospital in Tabora, Tanzania.

Special Challenges for Residents Going Abroad

Several national proposals have been made for trained U.S. medical professionals to serve abroad: a Global Health Service, consisting of a cadre of recently graduated physicians,[6] and "medical missionaries"[7] are just two of the groups involved. More and more residents are looking for international experiences during their residency years. An increasing number of formal and informal relationships are being created between U.S.A. and foreign governments, NGOs, and medical schools. While some are multilateral, most are unilateral, and they are as diverse as the countries and communities in which they are located. But while the daily duties may vary, the ethical issues are universal and unique to medical residents. Unlike medical students, who also frequently travel abroad to do short rotations to observe and learn, residents are more likely to examine and treat patients or be in the position to make clinical decisions in a foreign setting. Residents therefore carry a greater ethical burden since they may find themselves treating patients in situations that might demand clinical skills and experience they have not yet acquired.

The financial burden placed on a developing country by emigrating physicians, the governance of the growing international health workforce, and the volatile issue of the "Brain Drain" are increasingly coming under global scrutiny. Certainly in the years to come there will be greater regulation and oversight regarding the competencies demanded of residents from resource-rich countries practicing abroad.

If the in-country training physicians (medical and surgical residents) are required to demonstrate minimum competencies and obtain national registration before they are allowed to practice in their country, should U.S.A. residents be required to meet the same criteria before practicing in that country?

Should guidelines be developed for establishing "best practices" for working overseas?

An Evolving Perspective of Medical Ethics
Primum non tacere~ Above all, Do Not Remain Silent...

Delese Wear, Ph.D., Associate Director of the Human Values in Medicine Program at Northeastern Ohio Universities College of Medicine. challenges us to take advantage of 'teachable moments' in medical education and have the courage to speak out. She proposes another medical ethics mandate: *Primum non tacere~,* "Above all, do not keep silent."

Most of us acknowledge that global health experiences are personally transformational, leaving medical students and service providers with more than they could ever give. Global health education can be a great stimulus for modeling professionalism and cultural humility. It can lead residents to explore new ways of viewing the world, engage with different values, and motivate them to give meaning to their actions, process difficult feelings, and connect to their inner wisdom. Challenged by the uncertainties of life outside their comfort zone, residents often become more reflective and compassionate and develop a deeper social conscience.

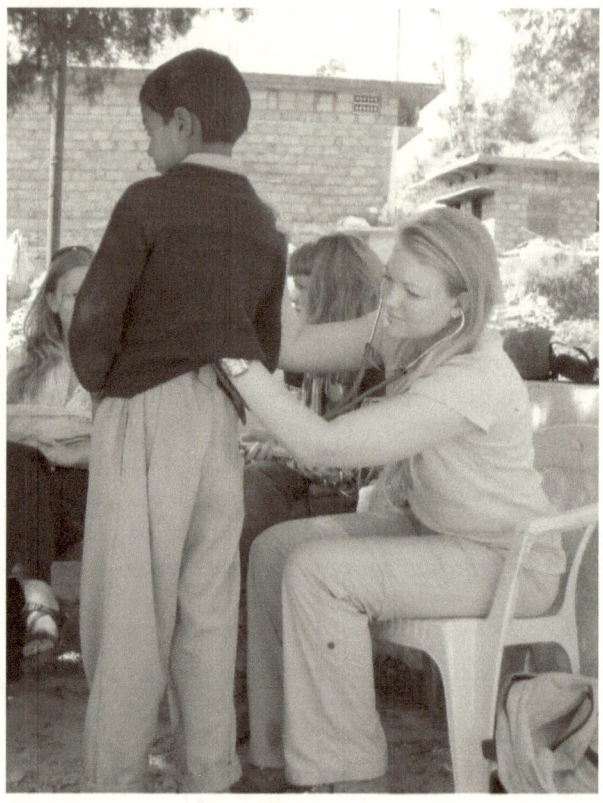

Child and Family Health International Rural/Urban Himalayan Rotation, alumna, with patient. During this rotation participants accompany a local physician, Dr. Paul, as he goes to surrounding villages to conduct health camps.

Physician Charter on Medical Professionalism

Applied to Global Health Ethics

In 1999, the American Board of Internal Medicine Foundation, the American College of Physicians Foundation, and the European Federation of Internal Medicine jointly created the Physician Charter on Medical Professionalism. It has been translated into six languages and endorsed by 90 professional associations, colleges, societies, and boards worldwide. It consists of three principles:

1. Primacy of Patient Welfare: Stresses altruistic dedication

to the well-being of the individual patient.

2. Patient Autonomy: Urges physicians to facilitate patient involvement in treatment decisions.

3. Social Justice: Calls upon physicians to work actively toward equitable societal distribution of health-care resources.

All three principles apply to the field of medical ethics. However, it is the third, social justice, which is especially relevant to the discussion of global health ethics. Because of the widespread social, economic, and human rights inequities, residents in training must be called upon to examine their reasons for going abroad and consider their responsibilities to others upon their return. A sense of personal social responsibility and a renewed intention to become a global citizen or agent of change can be the outcome of a global health experience.

Social justice examines the policies and practices (both formal and informal) relating to economic and political concepts of human rights and equality, health and welfare--"there is a general understanding that the voice of change should rise from the people."[9] This element of professionalism must be incorporated into any global health curriculum.

Dr. Alice Fornari, Ed. D. R.D., Assistant Director of Medical Education and Co-Chair of the Division of Education in the Department of Family and Social Medicine at Albert Einstein College of Medicine, suggests that in teaching social justice the point is for students to learn to question answers rather than to answer questions.

"By empowering our students and facilitating an environment in which they can think critically about medical issues, as well as medicine as a profession, we create future physicians who are empowered to think critically about social issues in general."

As residents plan their experience abroad, is it imperative that they have a true understanding of why they are going. Is it to provide medical care where there is none? Is it to learn new skills, such as cultural competency or a foreign language? Equally important, what will they do with the knowledge and skills they have learned once they return to the U.S.A. or other developed nation?

Questions that Prompt Ethical Discussion

1. What are your expectations about your formal education- what am I hoping to learn?

2. What are your expectations about your ability to provide health services- what can you give?

3. What are your institution's expectations about research and scholarly work?

4. Am I doing work that has been requested of the Residency or by the community?

5. Who gets the credit as the principal investigator if there is a publication?

6. Do you require local collaborators from the developing country to assist in writing?

7. What do you think/feel about medical tourism (where people go from one country to another for health care/procedures)?

8. What do you think/feel about medical education tourism (where trainees go abroad for a short time and spend part of it vacationing)?

9. How have social determinants affected public health of the community or particular region of the world that I am living/working in? How could you effect change?

10. Will understanding the historical, political, religious, and economic impact of the United States political policies influence my current and future work?

11. How can you support the goal "15 by 15", which aims to direct 15% of overseas funding toward professional development of the community workforce by 2015?[10]

12. How can you support the 15% Solution, in which medical journals devote 15% of their pages to issues in the developing world?[11]

13. What are community-based research initiatives? What did the local people ask of you?

14. Are my actions sustainable? If not, how can I make them so?

15. How is my presence affecting the local workforce?

16. Are the inequalities a result of the overarching system or of certain individuals?

17. Who is to blame? Who do you perceive has let the system down?

18. What is my role in perpetuating these realities of inequity?

Creating Your Own Recipe for an Ethical Residency Experience

This section may help residents select or create a global health rotation that takes into consideration the ever-expanding challenges. It is an attempt to stimulate thought and discussion in an area that may be evolving faster than the ethical principles and restraints that should be applied. The following series of suggestions are intended to help residents or faculty members design a rotation that is sensitive to the needs of the host site.

 1. Evaluate the out-of-pocket costs to the community and prepare to cover costs of training and education. At a minimum, reimburse hosts for the professional time and resources used and practice transparency and accountability.

2. Review personal and professional expectations and see if they align with the community's resources and expectations._

3. Be knowledgeable about the political, economic, social, and structural realities of the location to which you are going.

4. Do not practice beyond your means. As a medical student the

rotations are primarily observational, but residents will be asked to do something because they are the only ones available. Working in another country with patients is no different from home: use common sense!

5. Do not displace local health practitioners. Work side-by-side, offering relief and support when required.

6. Create partnerships that clearly benefit the community and are not demanding of its personnel or material resources.

7. Give priority to community participation and focus on projects that seek sustainability, i.e.: value professional development and training, not service and dependency.

8. Use appropriate technology and employ local evaluation metrics.

9. Be critical of research projects. Your responsibility is to function as an agent for the community and a guardian of their resources. Closely analyze the cost- benefit ratio of education and research. What sort of scholarly work is requested or required by the sending institution? Remain skeptical of the benefits promised.

10. For every service component or project there must be aspiration for systematic advocacy for change on a larger scale.

11. Be mindful of unintended consequences. Record facts and learn from them.

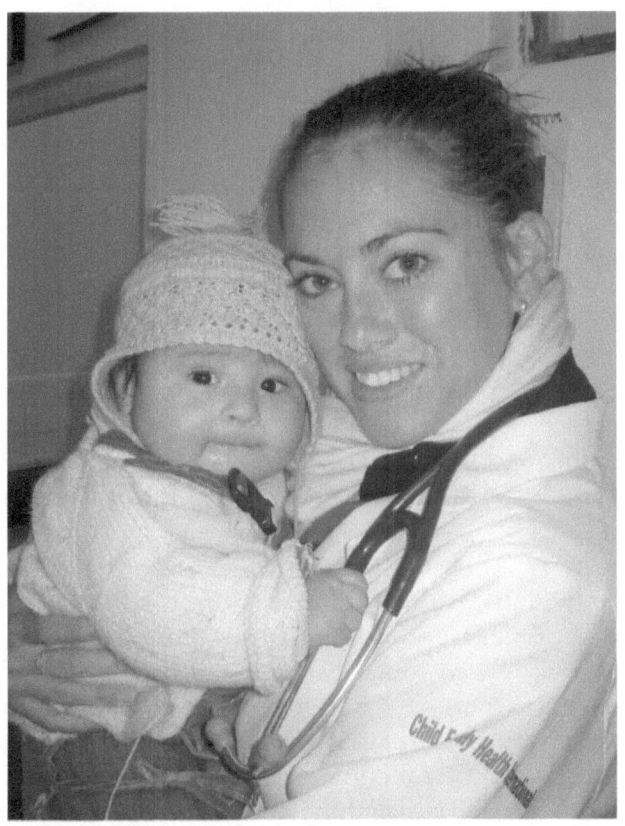

Child and Family Health International Pediatric Health in La Paz, Bolivia
alumni Ashley Strobel during rotations in Hospital del Niño, one of the largest
and oldest hospitals in Bolivia.

Incorporating Research into the Residency Global Health Program

The literature on ethical standards of practice involving medical research in developing countries is extensive. Community engagement and training, upholding IRB policies and protocols, authorship and ownership of intellectual property are all subjects that involve ethical considerations. Residents working abroad may have opportunities or even requirements to conduct research, often funded and directed by faculty at their academic institutions. Several questions arise:

1. Does doing research pose a conflict of interest with the goals of service and education for the resident in training?

2. Can the resident's short-term (generally 1-2-month) stay in the international setting offer sufficient time and experience to collect meaningful data?

3. What responsibility does the Residency Program bear in educating the local community about the pros and cons of the research?

Family Health International (www.FHI.org) has done an excellent job in teaching the local communities in developing countries the difficult and often abstract concepts of research ethics. A glance at their curriculum would be most helpful if your rotation includes any aspects of research. The ideal situation is incorporation by your Residency Program of its research agenda into projects designed and directed by the community partners and whose principal investigators are the local health officers.

Practical Applications for Global Health Ethics

Case scenario 1 --You are planning to go for one month to a rural health clinic in South Africa. You have been told that there is up to a 45% rate of Multiple Drug-Resistant Tuberculosis in patients diagnosed with HIV/AIDS. When you arrive with your two special filter masks, you feel guilty that you have not given your second one to the local physician. After putting the mask on, you experience embarrassment as the patients and family members giggle when you walk up to their bedside (the masks look like those the streets sweepers wear). The attending physician explains that no one wears masks at this clinic, not the health workers, families, or patients. You decide after a few hours to take the mask off.

●Should there be a policy that all practitioners from your residency program must wear the mask at all times?

●As the Residency Director of this overseas global rotation, is it okay to allow the resident to work without wearing the mask?

●Should the trainee sign a waiver of responsibility for the institution if he or she decides not to wear the mask? What if the trainee was a medical student or a pre-med student?

●What policies are in place at the local institution for

34

maintaining adequate cross-ventilation? If none, how can
you bring this to the attention of the administration?

●If every foreign student who came through the rural clinic
wore a mask, could it eventually affect policy change at that
location?

●Should your residency be willing to provide everyone masks
at the clinic if there was a mandatory policy that all U.S.A.
trainees wear them?

Case scenario 2 --You are beginning your second year of residency.
It is your first day of pediatrics in the Amazon Jungle. After an 8-
hour hike to a distant village you are told that the regional doctor
is out of the area on an emergency. The village health worker with
whom you were to be training has taken a month's vacation because
she heard another doctor was coming. You signed a residency contract
stating that you would not provide clinical care that was beyond your
means. You speak a little Spanish but none of the indigenous dialects.
Now there is no one to guide you but there is a ham radio that works
intermittently, used mostly to call planes in for emergencies.

●What would you do? What wouldn't you do?

●Would it make a difference if you were at a different stage in
your residency?

●Would it make a difference if you were fluent in the local
dialect or had a competent interpreter at your side?

●Is it fair and reasonable to get credit for a month of training
when there is no one there to evaluate your competencies?

You decide to stay and end up having a highly successful month
functioning as the local village doctor. No catastrophes occur and you
leave with the villagers surrounding you with great appreciation. The
village health worker returns along with the regional doctor thanking
you for your service.

●What would you tell your residency director about program
administration?

•Would you recommend this site for other residents?

•How would you define your role there, principally as a learner or as a provider?

•What recommendations and/or restrictions might you suggest for future volunteers?

•Would it be different if you were presented with the same circumstances but the rotation took place in the tundra of Alaska, north of the Arctic Circle? Why or why not?

Case scenario #3 --You are visiting a well-funded ARV Treatment Center in sub-Saharan Africa. You overhear a comment by a patient that 'it would be better to have AIDS because then I would get better medical care". You hear a story about a patient who seemed to have opportunistic disease symptoms, was hospitalized for a week, but then quickly discharged with a large bill when the HIV test was negative.

•What can you say to the patient? Do you tell the administration what you overheard the patient say?

•How can you find out if the story about the billing criteria is an accurate accounting of the situation?

•What actions could you take to change the policies that have led to this reality?

•How would you discuss this apparent conflict between lack of basic health care and specialized clinical services with your colleagues back home?

Case scenario #4 --You travel all the way to South Africa to participate in an NGO's Child Survival Project and learn that you can only see patients as a practitioner if you obtain the appropriate registration/ permit. You hear that it typically takes 6 months to get this approved. The clinic sees over 100 patients a day and needs you. You decide to work there anyway, seeing patients that otherwise would not get any care if you weren't there.

•Is this decision and behavior unprofessional? What could be the harm? What could be said in your defense? Can you identify potential value differences?

At the end of the month you realize that the experience does not fulfill the academic guidelines and requirements of your Residency Program

•Would you ask for special consideration anyway?

•If you are going to continue to receive your monthly salary, how are the funds distributed? Is the overseas faculty also getting paid?

Remember, the cultures, the inequities, and the absolute poverty of manpower and resources can undermine even the best prepared resident.

Summary

Global Health ethics can be discussed within many theoretical frameworks: human rights, governance and policy, technology and economics, and freedom of communication. The complexity and interrelationships of these concepts challenge even the most experienced clinicians and should be included in the training and preparation of residents working abroad. If we can create a flexible framework for Global Health Residency Training that responds to the voices of all partners, here and abroad, and if the program strives for moral decency, there is room for action. Certainly, if we have a greater understanding about how different systems affect areas of health care (access, distribution of resources, equity), the more applicable will be the solutions, the more sustainable the impact, and the more likely we will be able to function not only as service providers but as agents of change sowing seeds for political reform. Any global health program should develop and expand the individual's attitude toward the world and his or her place in it.

"The health of an individual may depend on particular susceptibilities; the health of a population depends on justice." -- *James Dwyer*

These concepts can be best taught/learned through a curriculum that values honest and continual reflection and questioning. We, as practitioners, must be willing and able to speak out and take action on the political, economic, religious, and structural realities that have influenced the vast divide between our own reality and that of the communities in which we serve during our short time abroad. These notions are articulated in Carl Taylor's new version of the Hippocratic Oath.[12]

"We must maintain the awareness that what we are doing is good, but it is not sufficient. Service can be a vehicle for awareness; it provides knowledge that there is more to be done to bring change in the larger systemic 'machine'." *--Rob Reich, Prof. Political Science 133, Stanford University*

Advocacy and activism are not expected or easy in the current western medical model. You may experience marginalization by speaking out.

In "What I Learned in Medical School", Karen Kim describes being labeled a "revolutionary," "social activist" and "communist" for her concern about disparities in health care, racism in medicine, and reforms in the medical system. "What is . . . disturbing . . . is precisely how little politicization and social consciousness it takes for someone in the medical field (even a student) to fall outside the professional mainstream."[13]

But we encourage you, as Gandhi so eloquently stated, *"Be the change you wish to see in the world."*

Other Useful Resources

For a comprehensive and thought-provoking review, we recommend 'Global Health Ethics' by Anvar Velji and John H. Bryant in <u>Understanding Global Health</u>.[14] Their chapter incorporates a holistic approach to the theory and practice of many diverse fields, including public and population health, biotechnology, scientific research, philosophy, anthropology, sociology, economics, religion and law.

The Virtual Mentor (American Medical Association Journal of Ethics) published an entire issue in December 2006 on the Ethics of International Medical Volunteerism and is worth a review.[15]

PLoS Medicine (www.plosmedicine.org) included four chapters detailing the ethical, social and cultural issues that are emerging from lessons learned from the Grand Challenges in Global Health Initiative. This is a 'must read' for any residents participating in programs that are funded by the Gates Foundation.[16]

The Advisory and Working Groups on Ethics through Community Campus Partnerships for Health (http://www.ccph.info), a non-profit membership organization that promotes health through partnerships between communities and higher educational institutions, is an excellent resource.

For more information on institutional governance and ethical standards, contact the International Consortium for Research on the Global Health Workforce (www.ich-ghw.org).

Carl Taylor's New Version of the Hippocratic Oath (1966)

I will share the science and art by precept, by demonstration, and by every mode of teaching with other physicians regardless of their national origin.

I will try to help secure for the physicians in each country the esteem of their own people and in collaborative work see that they get full credit.

I will strive to eliminate sources of disease everywhere in the world and not merely set up barriers to the spread of disease to my own people.

I will work for understanding of the diverse causes of disease, including the social, economic, and environmental.

I will promote the well being of mankind in all its aspects, not merely the bodily, with sympathy and consideration for- a people's culture and beliefs.

I will strive to prevent painful and untimely death, and also to help parents to achieve a family size conforming to their desires and to their ability to care for their children.

In my concern with whole communities. I will never forget the needs of its individual member

Reprinted with Permission

References

1. Declaration of Alma Ata, International Conference on Primary Health Care, Sep 1978, WHO Publication.

2. Strauss R. "Too Many Innocents Abroad" NY Times, 1/9/08. (Op-Ed)

3. Dodd C. "Expand the Peace Corps" NY Times, 1/14/08. (Ltr to Ed)

4. Garrett L. The Challenge of Global Health. Foreign Affairs Jan/Feb 2007

5. Pillar C, Smith D. "Unintended Victims of Gates Foundation Generosity" LA Times 12/16/07.

6. Stencel C, Vines, V. A Peace Corps for Global Health. In Focus. Summer 2005:5(2).

7. Panosian, C, Coates, T. The New Medical "Missionaries" – Grooming the Next Generation of Global Health Workers. NEJM 2006 354 (17):1771-1773.

8. Wear, D., in Professionalism in Medicine: Critical Perspectives. Wear D, Aultman, J editors; Springer Science, 2006.

9. Stern, D. Measuring Medical Professionalism. Oxford University Press, 2006.

10. 15 by 2015. Campaign partnered by GHETS, WONCA, The Network:TUFH, et al. Website: www.15x2015.org

11. Shaywitz DA and Ausiello DA. Global Health: a chance for Western physicians to give and receive. Am J Med. 2002 Sep;113(4):354-7.

12. Taylor, C. CS Ethics for an International Health Profession. Science 1996 Aug 153(3737): 716-720.

13. Kim K. in What I Learned in Medical School:Personal Stories of Young Doctors. Takakuwa, et al, editors. UC Press, 2004.

14. Understanding Global Health. Markle et al, editors. McGrawHill/Lange Medical, 2007.

15. Virtual Mentor: AMA Journal of Ethics. Dec 2006 8(12).

16. Tindana PO, Singh JA, et al. Grand Challenges in Global Health:Community Engagement in Research in Developing Countries. PLOS Med 2007 4(9): e273.

Acknowledgements: E. Gonzalo Claure Medina, Supervisor Outreach Program, Centro Boliviano Americano, La Paz, Bolivia: Dr. Wilfrido Torres Alvarado, Director of Regional Health for the Indigenous Nations of the Amazon,Puyo, Ecuador; Dr. Waman S. Bhatki, Joint Director (Training and Surveillance) and Monitoring and Evaluation Officer (GFATM/PPTCT), Mumbai District AIDS Control Society, Mumbai, India.

Chapter 4

Profiles Of Existing Global Health Residency Programming

A variety of residency programs have been established in global health, some formalized tracks, others less structured. This chapter presents a sampling of these programs to give readers an idea of program structure, challenges, and further resources for developing or expanding curricula.

Rainbow Babies and Children's Hospital Pediatric Residency International Health Track

Year Established: 1987

Location: Cleveland, Ohio

Disciplines: Pediatrics and Internal Medicine/Pediatrics

Website: www.uhhospitals.org/tabid/689/Default.aspx

Distinguishing Features

The Rainbow International Health Track program attempts to provide a component of global health teaching to any Pediatric or Medicine/Pediatric trainee who wants to participate. It is inclusive: you can participate regardless of your level of expertise. Among its purposes is to convey the importance of learning global child health issues as part of pediatric education in the 21st century.

•*Monthly lecture series:* The international health track program has a 2-year curriculum with lectures throughout the year. Topics include infectious diseases, epidemiology, nutrition, neonatal care, humanitarian emergencies, international research, the role and impact of NGOs, ethical issues and others. The global health lecture series are integrated into the residency program and all residents attend.

- *Journal Clubs:* There are 4-5 journal clubs per year. Residents and faculty participate in the article selection. Junior or senior residents present the articles and lead the discussions.

- *Electives:* A defined and pre-approved project of 4-6 weeks with pre-elective preparation and post-elective reports. In recent years several residents, particularly those who have been involved in global health before joining our program, have made two or even three trips during their residency or extended the duration of their elective abroad, using vacation time, electives, etc.

- *Elective Preparation*: Residents are required to go through a pre-trip orientation. They each get the assistance of a faculty mentor who is familiar with the area and can provide guidance. Residents preparing an elective abroad also get assistance from the global health education coordinator to cover practical issues, medical concerns, and liability issues. In addition, the program offers an annual course on "Preparation to International Health Service" that is highly recommended for residents planning electives abroad.

- *Faculty Mentoring:* As much mentoring as is needed is provided on a one-to-one basis. The program has a core of six global health faculty, as well as additional mentors in Family Medicine and Behavioral and Developmental Pediatrics with extensive experience abroad, who participate in mentoring of residents. Some residents have more than one mentor to cover different aspects of their elective. Residents also get advice from other residents who have been traveling to similar sites. The GH administrator offers guidance on all practical aspects of the trip and administrative requirements.

- *Presentations:* Residents are required to provide a report and a short presentation to the entire department. Some residents may be asked to present to a smaller group if numbers make it impracticable to present to the whole department. Some residents have presented their projects and/or research at national conferences.

Program Goals

The International Health Track program at Rainbow Babies and Children's Hospital was established by Dr. Karen Olness in 1987, with the following goals:

- Providing high-quality global health training for pediatric residents.

- Nurturing global health interests among the residents and broadening their career horizons.

- Providing experiences to help residents to develop sensitivity to health disparities and their causes, including health, social, economic and environmental factors.

- Provide experiences in child health epidemiology and public health, which contrast the child health situations in the developed world with those of developing countries.

- Providing clinical experiences to help residents improve skills in cross-cultural pediatrics in the United States.

- Providing a forum for diverse research opportunities in clinical medicine, medical education and impact on the workforce.

- Training advocates for children across the globe.

- Continually improving an innovative, nationally recognized model for resident education in global health.

- Developing pediatrician leaders in global child health.

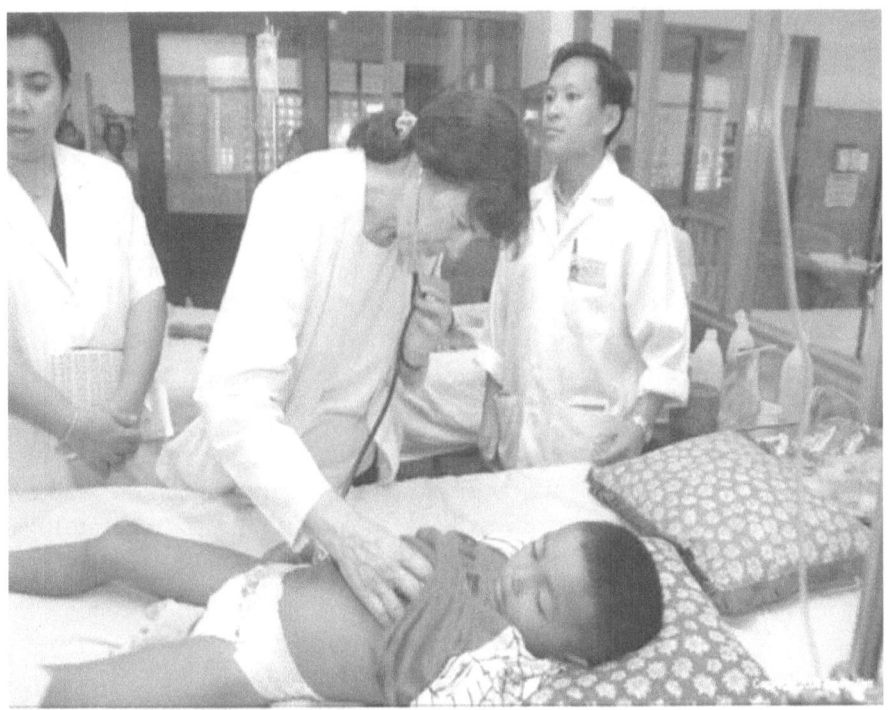

Karen Olness, MD, Founder of the Rainbow Center for Global Child Health and Rainbow International Health Track, in Vientiane, Laos.

Enrollment: Residents can enroll in the International Health Track at any point during their residency; however, the majority of them do so during PGY1 or early during PGY2. Currently about 60 residents (out of 90 in the program) are enrolled. Residents who complete an overseas or domestic international health-related project as well as the general curriculum requirements will receive a certificate of completion at the end of their residency training.

Additional Opportunities

- *Course:* "Preparation to International Health Service": Provided weekly from September to December. Strongly recommended to all GH residents – 18 hours total.

- *Course:* "Management of Humanitarian Emergencies: Focus on Children and Families". This unique and intense week-long course is recommended to GH junior and senior residents interested in pediatric disaster response – 40 hours total.

•*Research:* Owing to the limited time provided for most electives and the complexities of international clinical research legal requirements and ethical considerations, research is not encouraged, unless a resident has been involved in a project before the elective and complies with Institutional Review Board, etc. However, at times residents who had a special interest in research have worked with international research projects led by the GH faculty both at home and abroad; and others have been included in a research project that was already in place with a proper Institutional Review Board at the elective site. These types of electives usually require a greater time commitment and more personnel preparation.

•*Joining faculty in unanticipated opportunities.* Residents have had the opportunity to join faculty traveling to disaster areas. Some residents have also been involved in teaching in disaster trainings programs in international locations.

Management and Support

•*External Linkages:* The program has various degrees of relationships with the International Pediatric Association, Global Health Council, UNICEF, International Rescue Committee, Doctors Without Borders (MSF), World Health Organization, American Academy of Pediatrics Section on International Child Health, Red Cross and Red Crescent and Catholic Charities, particularly through the extensive work of Dr. Karen Olness in Uganda, Laos, and Thailand. In addition, the Rainbow Center continues to offer week-long training programs in disaster management geared to meet the special needs of children. These have been presented in the U.S.A. (14 programs offered in Ohio), Pakistan (three programs), Thailand (four programs), India, Ethiopia, Syria, Saudi Arabia, Panama, Nicaragua and El Salvador.

•*Funding:* The program receives some institutional funding for partial faculty support, one administrator and travel compensation for the residents who travel abroad ($1000/ person/elective). Several retired faculty contribute substantial volunteer time to this program. It also has received support from pharmaceutical companies who sponsor lunches and dinners during educational activities.

•*Program Management:* There are two co-directors of the Global Health Track and one half-time administrator; the latter is readily available to the residents, coordinates the educational programs, participates in recruiting, and serves as liaison with the global health faculty and the residency program.

•*Other Resources:* The GH program designs its own case studies. More case scenarios from collaborating programs would be highly welcome to enrich the pool of studies available. The program, which has been developing a bibliography, would welcome additional suggestions from other collaborating programs. Study guides and manuals are made available to the residents, particularly in the field of disaster management. We are receptive to all venues and opportunities to increase the amount and frequency of information that could be provided to residents, faculty, and all other professionals involved in global child health.

Program Outcomes

•Rainbow IH Track residents have done electives in 31 countries in four continents and have received scholarships and awards from organizations such as the American Medical Women Association, the American Academy of Pediatrics, and the MAP International Fellowship Program (formerly known as the MAP – Reader's Digest International Fellowship Program).

•Participating residents come from diverse backgrounds in terms of global health experiences. Pre- and post -tests are administered, and residents carry out evaluations at the completion of the program. Every educational activity provided is evaluated. Some interns are already knowledgeable and have received global health experience during their medical training. Many residents choose the Rainbow residency program precisely because of its global health program's reputation, its 20-year record, the depth of expertise displayed by the global health faculty members, administrators and volunteers, and their extensive accumulated experience in numerous countries, particularly in Asia, Africa, and Latin America. Incoming residents interested in global health are confident that they will receive all the support and mentoring they need, that the program will provide hands-on projects in the field, valuable additional learning opportunities and an integrated, flexible, and supportive program.

After graduation, these residents typically continue their careers with a strong international focus and dedication to GH. For other residents, this is an amazing discovery of the world beyond the United States. About half of the residents have never been outside the U.S.A. and/or grew up within very limited boundaries. When offered the opportunity to expand their horizons, some of them will open up and take advantage of invaluable experiences that transform them and affect their careers and personal lives. Graduates from the Global Health Track have gone on to work in just about every area of health care, including academic pediatrics, humanitarian aid, research, mission work, public health, child health advocacy, and private practice.

Contact Information:

Felicite M. Chatel-Katz, MA
Education Coordinator
(216) 844-8918

Marisa Herran, MD
IH Track co-director
Mherran2000@yahoo.com

Arlene Dent, MD, PhD
IH Track co-director
Arlene.dent@case.edu

Pediatric Residency Program; University of Washington (UW) / Children's Hospital and Regional Medical Center (CHRMC) Pediatric Residency GLOBAL Health Pathway

Year Established: 2008

Location: Seattle, Washington

Discipline: Pediatrics

Website: http://uwpeds.seattlechildrens.org/training/globalhealth.asp

Distinguishing Features

- Intensive 4-week curriculum involving case-based and local experiential training early in PGY2.

- This curriculum will include problem-based cases to cover global public health topics as well as an introduction to quantitative tools (epidemiology, basic survey design) to prepare them to design a Pathway Project. A menu of local clinical and community experiences is offered to residents, including work at immigrants/refugee children clinic; clinic for homeless adolescents; specialty clinics for tuberculosis, STDs, and HIV; local organizations serving refugee families, and community house-call visits with language/cultural translator to at-risk family home.

- Mentored Pathway Project conceived early in PGY2 and developed through the remainder of the second and third year. This Project will culminate in a paper and presentation that may be carried out individually or with a team of residents.

- Additional 4-week period in YR2 and 8-week period in YR3 to work on the Project activities and provide opportunities for off-site experiential learning.

- Structured career counseling, individualized learning plans, and mentorship for each participant

- Opportunity for Pathway and other residents to participate in a practical community-based health promotion elective involving a longitudinal partnership with a group called CHIMPS (Children's Health International Medical Project of Seattle) that serves the rural community of Abelines, El Salvador. This resident-run, faculty-supported collaboration with a community and local NGO (ENLACE) is an ongoing, sustainable, cross-cultural relationship that involves public health interventions and provision of sustainable medical care. It sends residents, faculty, medical students, and community pediatricians to this remote region to provide community-based health education during annual 1-week trips during the intern's vacation. This collaboration has led to evidence-based public health interventions that range from development of health educational talks for use by local CHIMPS members throughout the year to the provision of antihelminthic treatment, iron supplementation, and fluoride varnish supplies for administration by local health care providers. In addition, residents may travel for longer electives to work on specific projects with the NGO.

Participation: Residents apply to the pathways in the second half of their PGY1. The first cohort of Pathway participants was selected in 2007 and includes eight PGY1 residents in both the GLOBAL Child Health and Community/Advocacy Pathways (four in each pathway) from a class of 29. Residents interested in the Pathway but not selected for positions will have the opportunity to participate in the intensive curriculum as an elective, train overseas at developed sites, receive individualized mentorship and career counseling, and attend global health training integrated into the general curriculum (noon conferences, journal clubs, etc).

Program Objectives: The GLOBAL Child Health Pathway (GLOBAL: **G**lobal health, **L**earning, **O**pportunities, **B**uilding, **A**dvocacy and **L**eadership skills) of the UW/CHRMC Pediatrics Residency program endeavors to equip residents with the knowledge and experience to reduce health disparities and reduce the burden of disease among children in the U.S.A. and abroad.

The goals of the Pathway are to:

- Teach residents to recognize and address the impact of social, economic, environmental, and political factors on health disparities through experiential training and problem-based learning approaches.

- Provide practical public health and clinical perspectives on the management of health problems in resource-poor settings as well as best-evidence strategies for their prevention.

- Impart basic quantitative skills in epidemiology, study design, and biostatistics for evaluating and prioritizing strategies to reduce health disparities.

- Train residents to provide culturally competent, family-oriented health care for children as well as to communicate effectively and respectfully with health professionals within health care teams in international settings.

•Provide structured support to establish career paths for residents who plan to make global health a central part of their career.

Field experience: Participants in the GLOBAL pathways have an option to travel to other domestic sites or overseas in YR3 during the 8-week period. They may use this time to carry out their Pathway Project and gain experiential training. It is viewed as an opportunity for residents to apply the skills covered in the curriculum to community settings and to develop a network of professional and institutional contacts.

Established Sites: El Salvador, Kenya, and Peru.

Faculty: The two Pathways support a total of 0.5 FTE for dedicated Seattle-based faculty, as well as 0.5 FTE for a program coordinator. The residency program director is involved in the development of the program.

Funding: The CHRMC supports the faculty time dedicated to the Pathways development as well as a salary stipend for a number of residents to have dedicated time for global health training. Efforts are under way to seek further funding support for the Pathway activities. CHIMPS activities are supported through annual fund-raising and private donors.

Educational Materials: As part of the 1-month intensive curriculum, the Pathway program is planning to develop a series of cases that follow a problem-based approach. This case series would cover specific learning objectives by involving small teams of residents discussing and researching a series of pre-designed cases with a preceptor. These interactive cases include public health scenarios and aim to allow participants to gain and apply knowledge in global health topics, and exercise skills in epidemiology, health care administration, and cultural competency.

Monitoring and Evaluation: The learning objectives for the competencies will be evaluated throughout the residents' participation in the Pathway in order to assure adequacy of support for residents to fulfill learning objectives, utility of each learning objective for the resident career goals, and fulfillment of ACGME residency requirements. Individualized learning plans are to be developed for each resident specific to their interests, and reviewed periodically. Case-based self-assessments covering global health topics are being developed to help residents assess their confidence in these knowledge and practice areas. These materials are discussed with the resident's global health mentor, who provides guidance and support in meeting the resident's career goals.

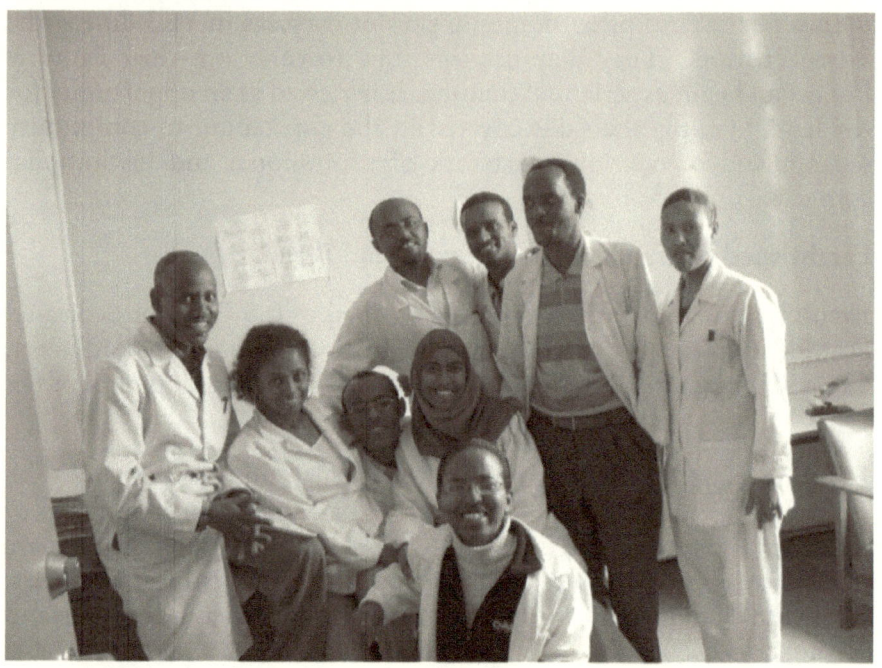

University of Washington resident Hiwot Hiruy (front center), with the B7 ward team in Black Lion, Ethiopia.

Challenges: Current challenges include the need to establish long-term funding to support resident travel and project activities. More support for junior faculty involvement with global health research and teaching is also needed to strengthen the program. Finally, effective means to ensure sustainability and reciprocity with overseas partners is a continuing challenge.

Future plans: Efforts are under way to forge greater collaboration with other programs at the University of Washington, including the Department of Global Health, through activities such as developing a conference for health professionals on the practical aspects of global health clinical work, sharing competencies and curriculum, and providing a structured cross-program faculty mentorship. Finally, there are also efforts to address the need to complete the continuum of global health education by providing support for training opportunities among clinical fellowships in the pediatric sub-specialties.

Other resources

Article: Suchdev P, Ahrens K, Click E, Macklin L, Evangelista D and E Graham. A Model for Sustainable short-term international medical trips. Amb Ped. Vol 7(4): 317-320.

Contact information:

Suzinne Pak-Gorstein, MD, PhD, MPH
suzinne@u.washington.edu

Elinor Graham, MD, MPH
ellieg@u.washington.edu

Heather McPhillips, MD
hmcphil@u.washington.edu

Mount Sinai School of Medicine Combined Global Health Residency in Medicine and Pediatrics

Year Established: 2007 (first class to begin July, 2008)

Location: New York, NY

Disciplines: Internal Medicine and Pediatrics

Website: www.mssm.edu/med-peds

Distinguishing Features

- Involves a four-year combined medicine-pediatrics residency in which graduates will be board-eligible in both disciplines and complete an MPH in Global Health. This program is part of a larger array of global health training tracks and electives organized by the Mount Sinai Global Health Center. It includes trainees from the departments of medicine, pediatrics, emergency medicine, obstetrics and gynecology, and psychiatry.

- Residents concurrently obtain an MPH degree with a concentration in global health that focuses on the health of disadvantaged populations.

- Residents spend 2-3 months doing fieldwork in an underserved community. They prepare a master's thesis and are expected to submit a paper for publication based on their work.

Background: Mount Sinai School of Medicine's Combined Global Health Residency in Medicine and Pediatrics is one of several global health training initiatives at the school, including global health tracks within the medical school and a Master of Public Health Program. Global health training for residents was launched in 2006 with an inter-departmental Global Health Residency Track. PGY2 residents from Internal Medicine, Pediatrics, Medicine-Pediatrics and Emergency Medicine were accepted into a 2-year program of didactics culminating in a 2-3 month field experience. In 2007, five residents graduated from this track. In 2007, the departments of Medicine and Pediatrics decided to introduce an advanced course of global health education, including an MPH in Global Health for residents entering the combined Medicine-Pediatrics program, resulting in the formation of the Combined Global Health Residency in Medicine and Pediatrics described below. The original Global Health Residency Track continues to offer training to residents in Internal Medicine, Pediatrics and Emergency Medicine, and since last year, residents from Psychiatry and Obstetrics and Gynecology as well.

Participation: All four of the entering residents annually participate in the global health program. Residents apply to the program as fourth-year medical students during the standard medicine-pediatrics recruitment season. Over 50 applicants were interviewed in the 2007-8 season for four slots. Residents are accepted into the residency program through the "match" process.

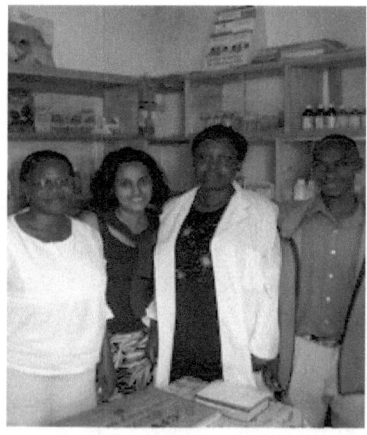

Mount Sinai Global Health Resident Dinali Fernando working to implement disease management algorithms in a rural Kenyan village pharmacy.

Program Goals

- To improve the health of underserved communities across the globe by training leaders in global health
- To promote the practice of evidence-based global health

Program Objectives: At the completion of the four-year residency program, the participating resident will have:

- Completed clinical training in both Medicine and Pediatrics and be board-eligible in both disciplines.
- Completed a Master of Public Health with a Global Health concentration.
- Developed the necessary knowledge and skills to adequately assess the needs of underserved and under-resourced communities.
- Developed the necessary knowledge and skills to design and measure the impact of interventions aimed at improving the health of such communities.
- Gained experience in implementation of research and/or public health programming in an underserved community.
- Completed scholarly work on a topic within global and submitted this work for presentation or publication.

Program Partners:

1. The Departments of Medicine and Pediatrics, which coordinate the participating residents' clinical training.

2. The Mount Sinai School of Medicine's Global Health Center, which provides overall program coordination, development, and administration.

3. The Mount Sinai School of Medicine's Master of Public Health Program, which provides the faculty and framework for the participating residents' global health didactic component.

Class work:

MPH course work requirements are completed during the four-year residency program. Classes are offered at night to accommodate resident schedules, and every effort is made to align heavier class loads with lighter clinical rotations. Residents take courses that are core requirements for the MPH, such as biostatistics and epidemiology, as well as courses that meet Global Health Core Competencies, such as Refugee Health, Health and Human Rights, and Maternal and Child Health. A number of specially designed seminars have been developed, including a career series, research meetings, and a pre-departure intensive skills workshop that also qualifies for MPH credit. Graduation from the MPH Program requires completion of 42 course credits, including a thesis.

Mentorship: During the first year of residency, residents are assigned a mentor with expertise in their area of interest. In addition to the Global Health Center (GHC) faculty, mentors are recruited from many departments within the medical institution and medical school. Colleagues from global health-related organizations in the New York area also participate.

Research and Public Health Projects: All residents are expected to complete a research or public health project during the course of their training. Residents begin the planning stages of their global health master's project in the first year of residency when they meet with global health faculty, identify a site and project, and are paired with a project mentor. Preparatory research, project methodology design, and initial data collection are encouraged during PGY1 and PGY2. During this time, residents present their projects to faculty and residents for review at regular research meetings. In PGY3, residents have 2-3 months of protected time to spend at their field site for completion of data collection or implementation of their project. On their return, residents are expected to produce a Master's thesis and a manuscript for publication. Additionally, they will present the results of their findings at a concluding seminar in their fourth year. They are encouraged to submit their findings for presentation at a national conference.

Fieldwork Experience: During the third year of residency, residents participate in a 2-3 month fieldwork experience as described above. (At present, the ACGME has approved only 2 months away from resident continuity clinic; however, a request for a 3-month exemption has been made.) Residents are strongly encouraged to perform their fieldwork research experience at a pre-approved site with which the GHC has an established relationship. Trainees and faculty from a few of these sites have already visited Mount Sinai for educational exchanges and such invitations will continue. Application for fieldwork research at a location other than a pre-approved GHC site can be made on an individual basis.

Faculty and Mentoring:

- There are five core faculty and a growing list of about 15-20 mentors from within the medical school and medical center, who are available to participating residents.

- A growing number of adjunct faculty from institutions and organizations outside Mount Sinai with specific areas of global health expertise (e.g., refugee health, disaster relief, human rights, health economics, etc.) also act as mentors.

- Core global health faculty salaries are partially supported by a philanthropic grant that funds the GHC. A salary line from the Mount Sinai Hospital also subsidizes faculty salaries in part.

Program funding:

- The Mulago Foundation, a private philanthropy group, supports about 75% of the overall Global Health Center activities. This residency program is one of several programs organized through the center.

- The remaining 25% is derived from other private donations as well as the aforementioned salary line and additional contributions from the Departments of Medicine and Pediatrics.

- The Departments of Medicine and Pediatrics cover MPH tuition expenses.

- Resident salaries are not interrupted while residents are away from Mount Sinai doing their field work.

- Travel to and from the field sites and living expenses while away are almost fully covered through the Global Health Center budget.

Program management:

- The global health component of the residency is currently directed by the GHC core faculty.

- The GHC has a full-time administrative assistant who helps administer all GHC activities, including this residency program.

The Department of Pediatrics has an administrator who also helps administer the residency program.

Monitoring and Evaluation:

- Residents will be surveyed regarding their global health knowledge, attitudes, and behavior at a few points during training, including at residency entrance and exit.

- Residents will be followed after graduation to evaluate the impact of their training on future career choices.

- Resident performance is formally evaluated at the completion of each clinical block and will be evaluated by their on-site supervisor at the completion of their global health field rotation.

- The global health curriculum and learning events are evaluated through written evaluations of each session and through resident focus groups.

Program evolution and direction:

- This is the program's first year. It is, however, a fusion of two pre-existing programs, the Medicine-Pediatrics Residency and the Global Health MPH.

Program challenges:

- Field sites – we have difficulty in identifying field sites that meet all of our criteria. In particular, it has been difficult finding reliable on-site mentors and appropriate longitudinal research projects.

- Residency Accreditation – At present, the program is considered a track within a traditional Combined Medicine-Pediatrics program. Therefore, residents are subject to many traditional requirements that limit the time they can dedicate to global health curricula and activities. Additionally, it has been challenging from the standpoint of both scheduling and receiving exemption from continuity clinic requirements to provide longer field work.

- Scheduling – This has been perhaps our greatest challenge in that residents in this program need to satisfy numerous requirements. Careful attention to the schedule is critical to allow for residents to dedicate appropriate time to each discipline of study.

External linkages:

- GHEC member

- We have organized the first meeting of a New York City area consortium of Global Health Educators and continue to promote collaboration among participating institutions through further events and online communication.

- We have organized an Annual Global Health Conference for the past several years. This year the conference will be co-sponsored by the regional GHEC.

- We have joined a consortium organized by the Earth Institute at Columbia University to improve health in Tanzania.

- We are engaged in a partnership with the Yale University School of Medicine's Global Health program to develop projects in Kampala, Uganda.

Useful resources:

- We undoubtedly will benefit from the growing number of online educational resources.

- Access to case studies in global health would also be very useful.

- We could benefit from additional medical education evaluation tools, specifically directed at assessing skills and knowledge of our global health residents.

- We would be interested in seeing models of waivers, memoranda of agreements, and contracts.

Availability of model documents: Model memoranda of agreements and insurance/liability forms are available upon request.

Contact information:
Jonathan Ripp, MD
Jonathan.Ripp@mountsinai.org

Brigham Women's Hospital Global Health Residency Program

Year Established: 2003

Location: Boston, Mass.

Discipline: Internal Medicine

Website: www.brighamandwomens.org/socialmedicine/gheresidency.aspx

Distinguishing features:

- Graduates can also receive an MPH from the Harvard School of Public Health. The MPH requires 6 months of classroom and campus study including July and August after PGY2 and PGY3 years, plus two January sessions. All MPH graduates must complete a project. Of the present enrollment about half are getting the MPH, one-third already have an MPH, and the remainder are pursuing other specialized studies.

- Program has strong links to overseas sites staffed throughout the year by several faculty as well as host country clinicians. The primary emphasis is on clinical care, providing residents a chance to develop excellent clinical skills as well as those relating to public health and program management. There are opportunities for residents to conduct research with faculty members overseas. The Haiti, Rwanda, Lesotho sites are affiliated with the Partners in Health NGO.

- Program emphasis is on promoting social equity and on getting residents to think more broadly about what global health means, domestically and internationally. Some residents elect to do field work in poor neighborhoods of Boston and may elect to work domestically on completion of the residency.

Participation: PGY1 residents apply in the fall for entry into the program in PGY2. Of the ~65 residents in the Internal Medicine residency, 11 applied in 2006 and 6 were accepted. The 2003 entering cohort completed their 4-year residency (3 years of which were in the global health program) in 2007.

Program objectives: The combined residency training program in global health equity and internal medicine seeks to:

- Provide clinical training in internal medicine that is culturally competent and promotes reduction of health disparities.

- Prepare physicians to address the impact of economic, societal, political, and adverse environmental factors on health status.

- Develop quantitative skills in public health, including clinical epidemiology, biostatistics, decision sciences, and health services research.

- Train future leaders in global/domestic health program

administration and advocacy, effecting change in health/social policy, and coalition building/funding procurement.

•Provide mentorship to trainees seeking applied and/or research careers in addressing health disparities.

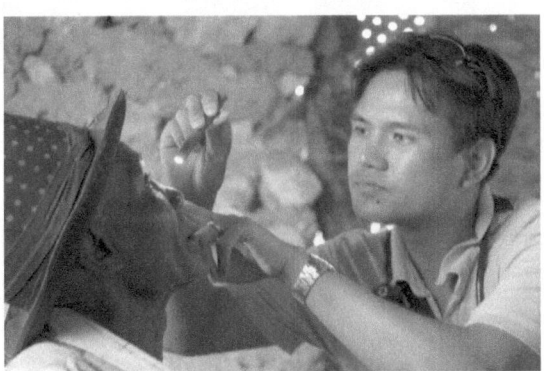

Photo by Matthew Lester for Partners In Health

Brigham and Women's Hospital Global Health Equity Resident Phuoc Le, MD, MPH examines a patient at a clinic in Haiti.

Curriculum: Global Health Equity residents complete a total of 48 months of multidisciplinary training including 3 years directly relevant to the subject. This expanded program fulfills the requirements for Residency Review Committee-Internal Medicine accreditation, as well as for an MPH. The curriculum includes training and education in global health equity, as well as the core competencies in internal medicine as defined by the ACGME. The program of study and field training includes the following:

•Clinical training in internal medicine, including ambulatory continuity clinic that is culturally competent and promotes reduction of health disparities.

•Overseas or domestic field work, research and coursework. All residents complete a project in one of three ways: a clinical research paper; a project leading to improvement in clinical services in their field site; or an evidence-based policy recommendations paper, preferably with publication. Those taking the MPH program have a required project.

•Preparation in addressing the impact of economic, societal, political and adverse environmental factors on health status.

- Comprehensive mentorship in clinical medicine and health disparities service and research.
- Graduate coursework leading to an MPH at the Harvard School of Public Health.
- Didactic seminars in global health equity and one internationally relevant conference or short-term training program per year.
- Longitudinal research in conjunction with Division of Social Medicine and Health Inequalities faculty.

The curriculum evolves as follows: PGY1, program application and acceptance; PGY2; a program orientation consisting of a group trip to a field site and one week of class instruction and 2 months of required rotations in Africa; PGY 3 and 4, 6 months of MPH instruction and 2-3 months in each at other sites. During PGY4 residents have the opportunity to serve as chief residents at a site and assume a major role as educators.

Field experience: Over the 3 program years residents spend most or all of 14 months abroad, reduced by 6 months if they do the MPH. Before assignment they receive necessary immunizations and briefings from the Traveler's Clinic. During the PGY2 residents are not licensed in the host country and hence must have their orders co-signed or overseen by a licensed preceptor. In PGY3-4 the residents obtain medical licenses in their host countries and thereafter serve as attending physicians. Residents may choose from among the various field sites that have been developed over the years by the Division of Social Medicine and Health Inequalities and Partners In Health. They include:

- *Zanmi La Santé*: serving a population of 500,000 in rural Haiti
- *Socios En Salud*: providing TB-related and primary care services in Lima, Peru
- *Partners In Health Russia*: providing TB-related services in Siberia, Russia
- *The Prevention and Access to Care and Treatment (PACT) Project*: providing HIV-related health promotion and harm reduction services in Boston
- *Equipo de Apoyo en Salud y Educación Comunitaria:* providing outpatient care to indigenous people in Chiapas, Mexico
- *Inshuti Mu Buzima:* providing services related to HIV, TB and malaria in Rwinkwavu, Rwanda

•*Bo-Mphato Litsebeletsong tsa Bophelo:* providing care to HIV and TB patients and women's health at multiple locations in Lesotho
•*Indian Health Service*: providing clinical services at sites in the Navajo Nation

Faculty: The program has two Boston-based faculty averaging half-time each plus an additional five faculty with lesser amounts of time. There are an additional four faculty members who spend most of their time overseas. The program director is 40% time and has the quarter-time support of a program manager and an administrative assistant.

Funding: A portion of the program support is obtained from BWH and Partners Healthcare, while the rest comes from fundraising, mostly individual donors. The program was launched with enough funds for 4 years and is now engaged in another fundraising effort.

Educational materials: Residents are asked to develop educational materials for their field sites and to make these available on the program's internal website. These include clinical teaching cases, photos, etc., for the more frequent clinical problems encountered. Most field sites have good internet connections and can access information on specific diseases and from such sources as the MSF handbook and WHO guidelines. The program, in partnership with the Harvard SPH, is considering developing teaching case studies similar to what has long been done by the Harvard Business School and others. Several faculty are now working on a case-based book for use by the residents and, after field-testing it for a year or two, may edit it for publication.

Monitoring and Evaluation: Residents are evaluated regularly by their supervisors in accordance with Brigham Women's Hospital and ACGME requirements, both while overseas and in Boston. At the end of PGY4 residents are asked for their overall assessment of the program and suggestions for improvement. Program faculty meet periodically to review program goals, methods, and accomplishments. Of the two graduates so far, one now works in the program and Haiti and the other is at the University of Pennsylvania working in pulmonary disease and MDR-TB.

Challenges: (1) Fundraising with the goal of becoming sustainable. This new program must turn away close to half of the applicants even though they are very well qualified. (2) Faculty: Creating sustainable career tracks for recent graduates and junior faculty. (3) Accreditation with the specialty Board: The main challenge has been to ensure sufficient continuity of clinic time, and residents have to adjust their schedule to comply with requirements. Good internet access from an overseas site allows residents to stay involved in the care of their clinic patients while away.

Future plans: The program would like to increase its capacity, subject to the ability to obtain additional and more stable funding. The number of potential well-qualified applicants greatly exceeds current capacity. The hopsital's Division of Social Medicine and Health Inequalities would also like to create a fellowship in global health to train physicians from other internal medicine programs and from other specialty residents.

Additional Resources:

Article, *Boston Globe,* 6/4/07: www.brighamandwomens.org/socialmedicine/News/Students%20called%20to%20global%20service.pdf

Article, *The Lancet,* Vol. 363, May 29, 2004, Paul Farmer, et al: http://www.brighamandwomens.org/socialmedicine/GHEarticleDR.pdf

Contact information:

Amy Judd
Ajudd@partners.org

The Albert Einstein College of Medicine/Montefiore Primary Care/ Social Internal Medicine Program Curriculum in Global Health

Year Established: 1970

Location: Bronx, NY

Disciplines: Social Pediatrics, Family Medicine, Primary Care Internal Medicine and Categorical Internal Medicine

Website: http://www.aecom-montefiore-medres.org/special_programs/social/curriculum.html#H

Distinguishing Features:

The distinguishing features of our global health curriculum and of our program, the Primary Care/Social Medicine Program in

Internal Medicine of Montefiore, are the synergy of "domestic" and "international" global health themes within a rich three-year curriculum; the emphasis on education in the context of service, contribution and capacity-building, as reflected in our actions in the South Bronx and Uganda; the depth and breadth of Einstein's faculty in global health; and the long-standing commitment of our hospital, Montefiore Medical Center, to the health of underserved communities.

Basic Program Elements

The purpose of the programs in Social Internal Medicine (since 1970) and Primary Care residency (since 1976) at Montefiore is to produce, in an academic environment of innovation and commitment, clinicians and physicians leaders who are equipped to improve the health of society, particularly among underserved populations domestically and globally.

Objectives/Expectations: The objectives of the Global Health Curriculum are as follows:
- To develop outstanding clinical skills that can be applied in diverse resource-poor settings in both the developing and developed world.

- To provide both the intellectual and the experiential foundations of culturally-competent clinical practice.

- To better prepare our residents for roles as health care leaders by presenting an inclusive global vision of the biological and social determinants of health.

- To illustrate and appreciate health disparities in their broadest context and the synergy between domestic and global inequity.

- To develop skills in population-based research and community-oriented primary care that can be employed to effect social change and improve society's health.

The Program's interest and commitment to global health, essentially a natural outgrowth of its fundamental philosophy, has been a significant factor in its successful recruitment of outstanding residents.

Program Overview:
Our curriculum in global health is not a "stand-alone program", with a separate residency "match number", but rather a set of courses,

rounds, and experiential opportunities within the Primary Care/ Social Medicine (PC/SM) Residency Programs in Internal Medicine at Montefiore. While all residents in the PC/SM Programs are eligible for the global health opportunities described below (and 90% participate), there is room for about 20%-30% of the residents in our allied programs to join.

Residents apply to the SM/PC Programs in Internal Medicine through the national match; there are 10 positions available in these two programs, five in each. The two programs have been united over the past decade with a joint curriculum, a single faculty, and one director and see patients in the same ambulatory clinic; however, for administrative and historical reasons they maintain separate match numbers. *All applicants are urged to apply to both programs, as both are highly competitive.* Once enrolled in the (combined) PC/SM Program, residents choose the global health opportunities as "electives". Eighty to ninety percent of SM/PC residents elect to pursue the Global Health Course and the international global health experience.

How Global Health Fits In:

Since our program leads to Board eligibility in Internal Medicine in 3 years, the amount of time residents spend abroad in their training is limited to 2 months: most residents spend 1 month. However, global health themes and domestic global health experiences run throughout the home-based curriculum as described below. Completion of the 3-year SM/PC Residency earns one third of the credits towards an MPH at the Columbia School of Public Health.

Of the 33 months of residency training, residents spend 16 on inpatient general and subspecialty wards and in intensive care units; 12 months in "General Medicine (GM)" rotations; and 5 "elective" months. The GM months, which distinguish the PC/SM Program, incorporate ambulatory medicine practice in our South Bronx community health center (the Comprehensive Health Care Center), in the poorest urban congressional district in the country, largely immigrant) with a special academic focus that varies each month. Prominently emphasized themes include: Clinical Epidemiology and Research, Community Medicine/Community-Oriented Primary Care, global health, immigrant health, women's health, HIV-AIDS,

Human Rights/Liberation Medicine, substance abuse, Geriatrics, and Behavioral Medicine.

The Global Health Curriculum: The Program incorporates both international and domestic global health themes and experiences into its curriculum, distributed over the 3 years of training.

Domestic Global Health:

- **Highbridge-Montefiore Community Health Worker Project**: created and continued by SM/PC residents, this initiative trains a cadre of South Bronx community members to reach out to, educate, accompany, and facilitate access to care for immigrants in the South Bronx and Northern Manhattan.
- **OPEN-IT Clinic**: (Opportunities Pro-immigrant and Newcomer – International Travel). Our resident-trained Community Health Workers and link immigrants to the South Bronx with our clinic through the bimonthly OPEN-IT Clinic.
- **Immigrant Health (IH) Rounds**: before each OPEN-IT Clinic, 1-hour rounds are held focusing on the diseases, health systems, economics, politics, and cultures of the countries of origin of the patients scheduled for the OPEN-IT Clinic on that day.
- **The Human Rights Clinic** of the Montefiore PC/SM Program: Started through collaboration between the Monte PC/SM Program and Doctors of the World in 1987, this monthly clinic was one of the first in the nation -- and the first whose providers are residents -- to document international torture and care for its victims.

International Global Health:

- **Health, Human Rights and Liberation Medicine**: an eight seminar course offered during the October GM Month that explores the relationship between health and human rights both nationally and internationally.
- **Global Health Course**: This highly rated course, offered at the end of the PGY II during the June GM Month, is an intense immersion into the clinical, social, economic, and political realities of health in the developing world. It features 70 hours of seminars led by internationally involved faculty from the Albert Einstein College of Medicine (AECOM), the Columbia

University School of Public Health, and multiple NGOs. The course is a prerequisite for the field experiences described below.

- **Uganda, GH Field Experience**: In collaboration with Doctors for Global Health and AECOM, the PC/SM Program has developed a close relationship with a medical school and rural hospital in southwestern Uganda. PGY3 residents can elect to work for one month caring for patients on the wards and clinics of a severely understaffed district hospital in Kisoro, Uganda. For many, the experience has transformed their career direction and sense of themselves as physicians.

- **GH Research option**: For residents who have global health experience before residency, are likely to pursue a career in global health, and apply to the SM/PC Program stating their desire to get involved with global health research during residency, a second month abroad can be elected in clinical research. This research is carried out under faculty supervision and can take place either in Uganda or in another site in the developing world. The entire project is not expected to be completed during that one-month field experience. The field work is but one part of a multi-component project whose conceptualization, Institutional Review Board application, analysis, and manuscript preparation occur in New York.

A word about the field experience in Uganda: The PC/SM Residency Program is committed to serving underserved populations in the Bronx and abroad and to capacity-building in areas of need. Despite the wealth of international opportunities available through the work of AECOM/Montefiore faculty involved globally, the program has chosen to stay with and contribute to *one* site in Kisoro, Uganda. In this way, through the contributions of our residents, we are able to provide this understaffed rural facility with consistent staffing every month, organize an ambitious continuing medical education series for its physicians, clinical officers and nurses, and contribute to its local Village Health Worker Program. The experience has been universally acclaimed by all who have participated, and in the context of a 3-year residency has clearly met our educational goals.

Logistics: Orientation, Management, Support, and Funding. Pre-trip orientation is extensively provided during the GH Course at the end of PGY2, at special events during the year, and regularly with the global health Director. The GH portion of the residency has a designated Director of Global Health and an Associate Director, both of whom are supported administratively. Full salary for residents is maintained while abroad, and housing is provided. Residents only pay for their plane flight. The PC/SM Program is supported by a combination of teaching budget, clinical revenue, and grant funding. The curriculum is supported by educational funding through both teaching budgets (80%), and educational grant revenue (20%).

Expectations: All residents are expected to prepare, in collaboration with the global health Director, three talks on clinical topics relevant to a resource-poor environment, and present them to the Kisoro staff. Those eligible for and choosing the GH Research option, also prepare a research presentation and report/paper before graduation.

Faculty and Mentoring: At present (2007-08), the program has three core GH faculty, each of whom devotes 25%-50% time to global health curriculum and field activities, supported by the Program and AECOM. Beyond the residency program per se, there is a wide range of global health-oriented faculty who are members of the Global Health Center at AECOM. AECOM has a 30-year history of involvement in global health research, education, and capacity-building, now represented by 30 to 40 faculty members with international research and service projects – an extensive network of available mentors.

Monitoring and Evaluation: Both the residents and the GH Course are evaluated formally every year. Both the domestic and international curricula in GH are evaluated semi-annually at program retreats. All residents say that the curriculum and experience have been formative, and many graduates have incorporated global work into their careers. But for a program that selects socially-oriented residents, and from which over 80% of graduates choose to work with underserved populations, the independent impact of our curriculum is hard to assess.

Program Challenges: We face three major challenges:

- Expanding global opportunities per resident within a 3-year curriculum, i.e., spending more than 2 months abroad is difficult vis-à-vis accreditation and Graduate Medical Education funding.
- Although the Program is supported financially by both Montefiore and AECOM, providing the present GH experiences

and curricula takes significantly more faculty time than is supported.

- •Global health is becoming more popular among students and residents. We would like to be able to meet this rise of interest among residents in other Montefiore programs, but are unlikely to receive the additional institutional support necessary to expand, and available grants are few.

External linkages: Our program relates closely to the larger movement of global health education. Our associate Dean of Education at AECOM, Dr. Al Kuperman, was one of the founders of IHMEC, now GHEC. AECOM and the Montefiore PC/SM Program has two faculty (Dr. Smith and Paccione) on the present GHEC Board of Directors. Dr. Victor Sidel, the past-president of the APHA and involved in global health throughout his long and illustrious career is on the faculty of the SM/PC Program. Dr. Lanny Smith founded Doctors for Global Health (DGH), and Dr. Paccione was on the Boards of both Doctors of the World and DGH. Dr. Ramin Asgary of the SM/PC Program continues to work for Medecins Sans Frontieres.

Useful Resources: We have created our own curriculum in global health over the years with lectures, articles, syllabi, and case studies. However, we are planning to incorporate GHEC's modules in areas in which we are deficient, use the GHEC Bibliography, and develop more case studies drawn from our field experiences and the literature.

Contact information:

Hillary Kunins M.D.
PC/SM Program Director
hkunins@montefiore.org

University of Toronto Family Medicine

Year Established: 1998

Location: Toronto, Canada

Discipline: Family Medicine

Website: http://dfcm19.med.utoronto.ca/international/default.htm

Distinguishing Features:

- •Currently, developing a third-year residency in international/ global health with two positions

•Orientation provided by the Centre for International Health at University of Toronto

Total participants in program: One or two residents per year in PGY3 but anywhere from 10 to 12 for 1-month elective in second year of residency and five or six undergraduates who wish to do an elective or summer project in primary health care.

Established field sites: Brazil, Cambodia, Chile, Columbia, Dominica, and Ecuador.

Funding: No separate funds at present for travel. Most residents receive salary support from the Ministry of Health in Ontario and take the time as elective time.

Faculty support: Three or four core faculty, informal mentoring arrangements, outside support from the Centre for International Health at the University of Toronto.

Time residents spend abroad: Varies from 4 to 8 weeks

Description:
This residency program is currently under development. Although residents have been traveling abroad with global health programs since 1998 in the Department of Family Medicine, this arrangement is only now being formalized. Significant international health linkages have been created, mostly to Central and South America, providing opportunities that some residents have pursued. These linkages have focused on capacity building of primary health care professionals in Brazil, Chile, and Bolivia.

The program highlights the most common methodology of developing residency programs. An interested faculty member(s) develops global health programs, and the residency training components are added as an adjunct. The key is recognizing residents who are interested in global health and linking them with faculty members who are willing to support international electives in developing countries.

Family Medicine's core training in Canada is 2 years; a third year can be added to increase competency in an area. One of the areas that will be developed is global health.

There is funding for a program director, Katherine Rouleau, and a program assistant to help develop the residency and aid the director.

The program is currently seeking how to develop effective management and monitoring of its programs.

A new program in global health faces major challenges: difficulties obtaining university support and raising funds to develop a program, establishing field sites with appropriate counterparts, and finding time to develop curriculum components for an appropriate third-year program. However, even with modest means, successful programs can be established.

Contact Information:

Yves Talbot
y.talbot@utoronto.ca

Kathrine Rouleau
Rouleauk2002@yahoo.ca

University of Pittsburgh Global Health Program in Reproductive Sciences (GHPRS)

Location: Pittsburgh, Pennsylvania

Year Established: 2006

Specialty: OB/GYN

Website: http://obgyn.medicine.pitt.edu/content.asp?id=336

Distinguishing Features:

- International rotations of 4-6 weeks during the 3rd year of residency, with costs covered by GHPRS program.

- Well-defined curricular objectives.

- 3-year optional Global Health Track, including an 18-credit core curriculum leading to a certificate in Public Policy and Management.

- Residents participate in Global Health Seminar Series organized by the School of Medicine and Graduate School of Public and International Affairs.

Program Mission

To provide global health education to residents, fellows, faculty, and medical students in obstetrics and gynecology and the reproductive sciences while improving health care in the United States and developing countries.

Specific Goals

- To develop a collaborative link between international health care and domestic health care participant sites.
- To provide health care to underserved women.
- To collaborate in research aimed at improving the health care of women in developing countries.
- To enhance bi-directional clinical and research experiences for residents and faculty physicians in developing countries.
- To increase awareness of cultural differences and lifestyles that challenge underserved women's health care in the United States and developing countries.
- To encourage lifelong interest in global women's health among residents.

Program Curriculum Objectives:

- Know the Millennium Development Goals as they relate to improving women's health care.
- Understand strategies to promote reproductive health in other countries.
- Diagnose and treat diseases such as malaria, cholera, tuberculosis and parasitic diseases in women.
- Interact effectively with individuals from cultural backgrounds different from those of trainees.
- Recognize the differences in health care practices, beliefs, and expectations at the international site.
- Practice medicine in developing countries with limited resources.
- Contribute to the establishment of bi-directional clinical and research ties with the host country.
- Develop core knowledge, skills, and attitudes to maintain a lifelong commitment to global women's health.

Curricular Components:

Short-term International Experience

Residents may opt to spend one rotation abroad during their 3rd year. Residents unable to travel abroad for personal or family reasons may arrange an underserved domestic site experience. Residents are encouraged to start the planning process as early as possible by speaking with a faculty member of GHPRS no later than 6 months in advance. Residents will spend 4-6 weeks working at a designated site practicing obstetrics and gynecology. Trainees may be supervised by an attending from the University of Pittsburgh or by the collaborating site. The cost of travel, vaccinations, and (if needed) anti-malarial medications will be covered by the GHPRS. Medical students are invited to join residents and faculty mentors during a supervised international experience.

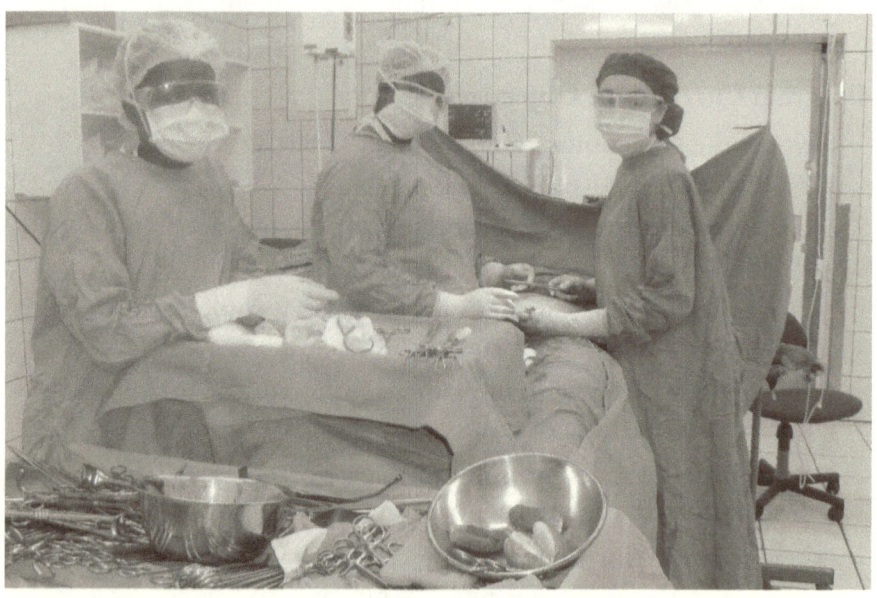

University of Pittsburgh OB/GYN resident operates with colleagues in Swaziland.

Global Health Track

The Global health Track is a three-year program offered to first and second year residents. It includes a core curriculum that leads to a certificate in Public Policy and Management: Global Health in

Reproductive Science. Two residents are selected per year (PGY-1/PGY-2) through an established application process. These residents receive additional support and "flex time" to complete required course work and participate in community and international rotations. Seminars are currently offered once a month in the evening and include all disciplines. Each fall, program coordinators will select two PGY-1 and two PGY-2 residents for the Global Health Track. They will be attend didactic sessions once a month during work hours. In addition to their international rotations, they will work in neighborhood clinics that serve the local indigent population. All these experiences are practicum-based with faculty mentoring that adhere strictly to Residency Review Committee guidelines. They must stay within the 80 hour/week requirement.

Collaborative Curriculum

The University of Pittsburgh School of Medicine and the Graduate School of Public and International Affairs (GSPIA) have developed a set of global health seminars that residents participating in the GHPRS program will be scheduled to complete. This collaborative program examines the challenges inherent in developing and sustaining improved health outcomes in developing countries. One of its primary goals is to familiarize physicians with the complexities and uncertainties of working in resource-poor environments and to provide a knowledge base and skill set to help practitioners overcome the many policy-related and institutional barriers to successful health outcomes. The program is designed to challenge conventional approaches to problem solving and decision making and alert professionals to the factors that impede the planning and implementation of effective, efficient and sustainable health policies and systems in developing countries.

The collaborative Global Health Program will offer 12 advanced seminars on global public health issues over the course of one year, beginning January 2008. Program participants include physician-residents pursuing the global health track in the School of Medicine, as well as upper-level medical students and working professionals interested in global health issues.

The seminars complement the global health curriculum and lecture series sponsored by the School of Medicine, and emphasize global health policy and practice from an international development perspective. The field of international development comprises a diverse range of global, national, and regional organizations that often partner with the governments of developing countries to provide funding, personnel, and expertise to reduce poverty and support health, education, and other programs. The program and curriculum design for the seminars were developed in collaboration with the faculty of the School of Medicine, and work with curricula in the following areas: the GSPIA's Masters of International Development, the Master's of Public Administration's major in policy research and evaluation, and several fields in doctoral programs.

The curriculum for the seminars focuses on five broad areas of concern for those interested in effecting policy change, health interventions, or health outcomes in developing countries:

- The political, economic, and socio-cultural context of health policy and health systems development and implementation in developing countries.

- The influence of corruption, low capacity, and weak governance systems on institutional performance and the achievement of health-related policies and interventions.

- The tools, techniques, and methodologies commonly used by international development organizations and global health institutions for identifying needs, designing interventions, and assessing health program and policy outcomes.

- An in-depth review and assessment of five development policy and practice domains with a significant health dimension: human rights, conflict and population displacement, gender, child development, and environmental crises and disaster management.

- A comprehensive review of obstetric and gynecological challenges incurred in limited work force and resource poor areas and their impact on the global society.

The Curriculum

A core group of GSPIA faculty will develop the syllabus for each seminar and facilitate the seminar discussions. Faculty members at the School of Medicine with an interest in global health are also expected to join the seminar discussions. The seminar topics identify the key themes in international development policy and practice. Their format is similar to GSPIA's doctoral seminars, where students synthesize and critique an extensive, diverse range of literature relevant to an understanding of perspectives and research methods that guide policy, program, and institutional design, as well as performance-monitoring and evaluation. Case studies also will be used to stimulate discussion, emphasize key themes from the readings, and engage students in planning and problem solving in diverse country settings, working with various sub-populations.

Faculty will supervise each student in choosing a country and developing a research topic for investigation over the year-long course of study. Students are expected to develop and present several short policy briefing papers, and to produce and present a comprehensive policy paper or research design by the end of the year. Upon completion of the year-long plan of study, students will have achieved the following learning objectives:

- Assessed the political, economic and socio-cultural determinants, which influence health policy and practice in diverse developing country settings.

- Demonstrated the application of diverse research and analysis tools and techniques used in facilitating problem solving and decision making in resource-scarce environments.

- Investigated the structural and systemic weaknesses that underlie many of the key institutional, regulatory, and governance mechanisms necessary for conducting and monitoring public health interventions and outcomes.

- Acquired a mastery of the complex problems and barriers to successful health outcomes for population groups such as women and children, and the challenges involved in health service delivery and management in situations affected by conflict, repressive governments, and environmental crises.

Medical Student International Rotation

A fourth-year elective in Reproductive Health in the Developing World is currently available. Administrative assistance is available to medical students but GHPRS will not cover direct expenses.

Strategic/Networking Plan

The GHPRS strategic plan is focused on six major process objectives. Networking with key faculty and personal, community leaders, and international partners will be essential to establish the following comprehensive components:

1. Curriculum development

2. Site identification that meets curriculum objectives

3. Established faculty mentorship program

4. Projected budget and long-term financial goals to establish financial sustainability

5. Formalized institution-to-institution clinical care and research collaborative memorandum of understanding

6. Evaluation and redesign

Faculty Mentoring: Fifty-nine full- and part-time faculty, as well as 18 staff physicians, volunteered to travel with residents. According to a University-wide survey, 15% of the OB/GYN faculty has international experience. On the basis of this survey and communications with faculty, the participating faculty was selected. In addition, four international sites were visited, memoranda of understanding were signed, and relationships with in-country mentors were established.

Funding: The prudent decision to develop a global health program stems from the recognition that all physicians must be trained as global physicians. Owning the health care challenges of the world as our own drives the strategies that promise to affect health care of both resource –rich and poor populations. Investing in medical education, the root of future growth of a people, community, and many nations must be part of a legitimate training program. Funding is provided by the Department of OB/GYN and Magee Women's Hospital. Funding from an anonymous foundation was also procured to support a collaboration involving specialty training in developing countries. It will include resident and faculty stipends. Creating a series of educational sessions while at the host site allows for CME credit and use of CME funds for volunteer faculty. Currently we are pursuing salary support for a fifth fellowship year for interested residents.

Contact Information:

Margaret D. Larkins-Pettigrew,MD,MED
Larkinsmd@upmc.edu

Yale/Johnson and Johnson Physician Scholars in International Health Program

Year Established: 1981

Location: Hartford, Connecticut

Disciplines: Residents from all specialties are accepted into program

Website: www.info.med.yale.edu/ischolars

Distinguishing Features

- Accepts ~50 physicians per year for 4-6-week rotations at hospitals in five countries. About half of the participants are Yale residents, one third come from other residency programs, and the balance are career physicians.

- Provides on-site mentoring by well-qualified nationals and intermittently by Yale faculty and senior career physicians.

Background: The Yale/Johnson and Johnson Physician Scholars in International Health Program at Yale Medical School offers international medical experiences for residents (and career physicians) from across the U.S.A. who are interested in building capacity by developing partnerships of patient-centered care and models of teaching in low-resource settings.

Sites: Sites have been established in Uganda, South Africa, Eritrea, Vietnam and Honduras and are being developed in Indonesia and Liberia. Certain sites provide the opportunity to take language classes and have the services of an interpreter when necessary.

Applications: Applications are accepted in January for the forthcoming academic year (July – June). (See www.info.med.yale.edu/ischolars.) A review committee, including an external reviewer, meets after the deadline to review applications; accepted scholars are informed in February. The Yale/ Johnson and Johnson program accepts about 50 physicians per year, about half of whom are Yale residents, one third are residents from other U.S.A.-based teaching hospitals, and the balance are career physicians. Participants may present a list of their top three choices for rotation. Career physicians are welcome to propose a rotation at an independent site, which will be subject to review to determine quality of mentorship and medical experience.

Logistics: Housing is often coordinated by the site. Participants are responsible for travel to, from, and within their site, in addition to food and lodging. To supplement these costs, each participant will be granted a reimbursement award, based on the site to which they travel. Salaries of Yale residents are maintained, as are malpractice insurance and workman's compensation. Pre-travel vaccination and a HIV ART blister pack are provided for Yale participants. Outside participants will need to satisfy pre-travel requirements at their expense.

Faculty and mentoring: Mentors at each hospital site, chosen by our directors based on personal relationships, provide first-hand experience for residents during rotations of 4-6 weeks. At times, Yale faculty and senior career physicians rotate with residents.

Program funding: Grant funds from two major foundations have been awarded since 2001 to support stipends for the selected applicants and to support the U.S.- based program management.

Program management: Dr. Michele Barry and Dr. Frank Bia are program Co-Directors. They are involved on a daily basis with program management. Full-time administrative coverage and support is available at Yale for the overseas mentors and scholars. An International Health Program committee composed of the program directors, staff, faculty, and chief residents meet regularly.

Monitoring and evaluation: Evaluations by the scholars of their experience and evaluations of residents by their mentors are required. The scholars' evaluations are shared with mentors to address weaknesses noted in the rotation experience.

Program evolution and direction: The International Health Program, started in 1981, focused on providing an international rotation at one of over 15 sites to Internal Medicine residents at Yale. It was created to offer overseas experiences for residents. Funding from Johnson and Johnson, obtained in 2001, has changed the focus to fewer overseas sites with an emphasis on capacity building in truly underserved settings. An evening course on the socio-political aspects of global health is offered throughout the year as an elective. We hope to develop a four-year MPH program in global health and global social inequities.

Program challenges
- Refunding annually (>25 years, but tenuous)

- Career pathways for residency
- Protected time for faculty to rotate to sites
- Finding money to develop an MPH Global Health and Social Disparities Residency track

External linkages: Michelle Barry is past present of American Society of Tropical Medicine and Hygiene, Chair of IOM Global Health Interest Group, and member of GHEC.

Useful resources: Gupta AR, Wells CK, Horwitz RI, Bia FJ, Barry M, 1999. The International Health Program: The Fifteen-Year Experience with Yale University's Internal Medicine Residency Program. *Am J. Trop. Med. Hyg.*, 61:1019-1023.

Contact Information:

Laura Crawford MPH
laura.crawford@yale.edu

St. Joseph's Regional Medical Center Family Medicine Residency Program

Year Established: 1990

Location: South Bend, Indiana

Discipline: Family Medicine

Website: http://saintjosephresidency.com/inthealth/

Distinguishing Features

- Residents allowed 2 sequential months of international elective time.
- Program pays salary and all travel/educational expenses of international activities.
- Community-based residency training with a domestic correlate of an underserved, multicultural patient population.
- Annual seminar series of 10-15 didactic lectures to augment global health experience.
- Graduates of program have created a non-profit Global Action Community, website www.sbglobalaction.com

Participation: About 40% of the annual class of nine residents participate.

Established field site: none

Funding: Annual program costs depend on the number of participants. Each resident's international rotation travel expenses and program costs are covered by the residency program. In addition, salary is maintained during up to 2 months of international rotation. Funding is provided by the institutional budget.

Faculty Support: One faculty has financial support and protected administrative time to coordinate the program. The seminar series is staffed by this faculty member, visiting speakers, and residents.

Time Residents Spend Abroad: Up to 2 consecutive months.

Curriculum Structure: The global health curriculum consists of a series of seminars that provide an overview of topics, such as malnutrition, the ethics of medical missions, and HIV/AIDS. These take place during protected didactic time. The resident's international activities are essentially independent activities. Residents are assisted in finding and evaluating potential sites by the faculty coordinator. The domestic population served by residents is underserved and multicultural, providing a natural correlate to global activities.

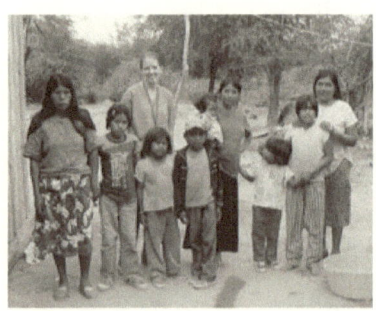

St. Joseph's Family Medicine resident rotating abroad.

Description

This global health track is open to all interested residents: usually about one-third participate. Most who participate have had global health experience. The program relies heavily on the interests and experience of a faculty "champion" who has protected time to administer the program. The mainstays of the program are a didactic series that provides an overview of information on a variety of topics and an international experience funded by the residency program. Each resident can take part in up to two international experiences for a maximum of 2 months. Most choose clinical experiences, while others prefer to do course work in tropical medicine or other relevant topics. Upon their return, residents are required to write an article for the program newsletter and present their experience at a noon conference. No research is required during the experience.

Anecdotal evidence suggests that residents respond positively to their experience. There is no formal evaluation mechanism or quality assurance. At international sites residents are overseen by a preceptor, who provides evaluation of their performance. St. Joseph's has found this program to be a good recruitment tool and a successful correlate to their local underserved, multicultural patient population.

The main hurdles identified by the program are its small size and having only one faculty member with dedicated time and an interest in global health. The program has not encountered Resident Review Committee problems nor any malpractice issues. No malpractice insurance is provided for residents rotating abroad. There is no formal orientation or debriefing for residents around their international experience. The program coordinator provides formal mentoring and attends relevant meetings of the American Academy of Family Physicians, Global Health Education Consortium, and Society for Teachers in Family Medicine. The residency program is currently expanding its global health track to offer a 4-year option that will include a Master in Public Health funded by the program.

Graduates of the program have formed the Global Action Community (www.sbglobalaction.com). It holds a monthly speaker series, organizes medical supply donations, and does direct patient care abroad.

Contact Information:

Kevin Ericson MD
ericsonk@sjrmc.com

Lawrence Family Medicine Residency Global Health Curriculum

Location: Lawrence, Massachusetts

Discipline: Family Medicine

Website: www.lawrencefmr.org/index.htm

Distinguishing Features:

- $60,000 annual investment in language training, including 10-day intensive Spanish course at Dartmouth College.

- All 1st year residents participate in a week-long visit to sister program in Dominican Republic for educational and cultural exchange.

- Structured longitudinal relationship and elective with Nicaraguan clinical site, including pre-departure preparation and structured mentoring.

- Full coverage of travel/tuition for additional language training during elective time.

- Domestic global health correlate with a predominately Dominican patient population at a community-based training site in urban underserved community 30 minutes north of Boston.

Participation: This year, all residents who enter the program annually participate in global health activities.

Established field sites: Nicaragua, Dominican Republic

Funding: The program funds approximately $60,000 per year in language training activities. In addition, it funds the annual intern trip to the Dominican Republic, a $500 annual Continuing Medical Education stipend, and support of language school training during elective time. In part, this funding is facilitated by the health system's passage of a relatively large percentage of training funds into the residency program.

Faculty support: Five of the 30 faculty members have substantial global health experience and act as informal mentors. Dr. Tony Valdini acts as program director and has salary support for his in-country work in Nicaragua as well as secretarial support at home.

Time residents spend abroad: 1 week during intern year in the Dominican Republic, and up 2 consecutive months during 3rd year elective time.

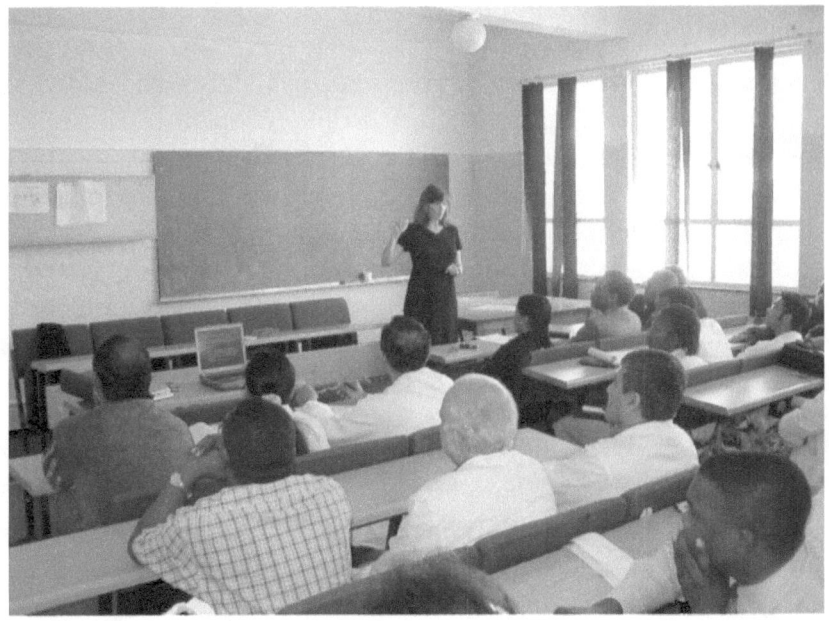

Lawrence Family Medicine residents Phil Bolduc, MD and Jen Reidy, MD teaching in South Africa.

Curriculum structure: There is a uniform curriculum for all residents during the intensive language training at Dartmouth College that precedes clinical obligations of the intern year. Subsequently, six to eight global health lectures are given per year in the core curriculum, provided by both faculty and residents with global health experience. Additionally, there is a structured program covering history, geography, culture, and health care provision over the weeklong exchange with a sister Family Medicine residency program in the Dominican Republic. The program accommodates the training goals of many residents by allowing flexible scheduling to complete additional field work or complementary degrees (e.g., MPH).

Description

Lawrence Family Medicine Residency's global health programming reflects the predominantly Hispanic patient population it serves in northeastern Massachusetts. According to Program Director Scott

Early MD, "In general it is a very customizable approach. There is no formal track that people enter." Despite the absence of a formal track, the program has a strong commitment to global health programming. Before initiation of clinical responsibilities, all residents go to Dartmouth College for the intensive language course. Throughout the remainder of the residency, group Spanish classes and individual teaching are available during protected time. A Spanish teacher even accompanies residents during clinic visits. Although residents are encouraged to use their Spanish, interpreters are available to critique and assist. The Spanish teacher also prepares and presents about 16 individualized one-on-one hour-length tutoring sessions for each first-year resident and is available to second- and third-year residents as needed. In total, $60,000 is invested per year on resident language training. Each first-year class travels to the Dominican Republic at the beginning of March, visiting a Dominican Family Medicine Residency, learning about the country's history and geography, and attending educational programming at the sister institution. While residents use vacation time for this trip, the residency program supports related travel costs. This experience helps residents relate to the largely Dominican population in their catchment area.

During their second and third years, residents are encouraged to take part in international electives. Approximately two-thirds of the average resident class of eight, takes advantage of this opportunity. Lawrence offers a structured elective through an ongoing relationship with a clinic in Nicaragua. This experience includes a faculty supervisor, pre-departure preparation, and a longitudinal context. Residents are allowed up to 8 weeks of international elective at one time. Their salaries are maintained during this period, and they may apply a $500/ year educational fund toward related expenses. If the international rotation involves attending a language school, the residency program will cover the cost of tuition and travel expenses. Usually this linguistic training is in Spanish, but it may be another language that will enhance the resident's ability to care for underserved patient populations. For instance, one resident went to a French-language school as she plans to work in West Africa after graduation. Most residents find their own international rotation site. The site and a local supervisor require approval by the residency program director. Upon returning, most residents choose to make a presentation on their experience.

Of Lawrence's faculty, almost two-thirds have at least some global health experience and a few have more than 10 years of experience. These faculty members mentor residents in an informal fashion. Although there is no formal evaluation of the mentoring or global health experience during residency, data are collected on the development of Spanish proficiency at five points over the course of the residency. This sequential evaluation shows an impressive increase in proficiency by residents.

The residency has a longstanding association with the NGO, Bridges to Community. Through Bridges, members of our community have worked in a health post in Mongallo in northeast Nicaragua. This group includes four present residents during their medical school careers, three faculty members, and several other current residents and graduates. This association continues.

While in medical school at Dartmouth, and after attending a Bridges trip, one resident, Dr. J.P. Dedam, founded a development NGO that serves the Mongallo area. This NGO, *Hermanos por la Salud*, is involved in agricultural projects, including a cheese factory and a pilot project in the breeding of pelibuey (short-haired sheep). The Nicaraguan members of the Mongallo co-operative have asked the residency to help them improve their facility and services at the health post; the Lawrence Family Medicine residency is in process of "adopting" the Mongallo health post along with its nurse and *promotores* (lay health workers). Ten residents are now involved in planning and implementation of the adoption process and creation of a year-round elective. This association will allow residents and faculty to work safely in a remote facility with known resources and they are supervised by faculty, the local MINSA physician, and usual health post nurse. At present, the residency staff working in Mongallo lives with a Nicaraguan family, which enriches the experience. Siuna, the largest nearby town, is an hour's plane ride from Managua. Mongallo is an additional 90 minutes by bus from Siuna or 12 hours by bus from Managua.

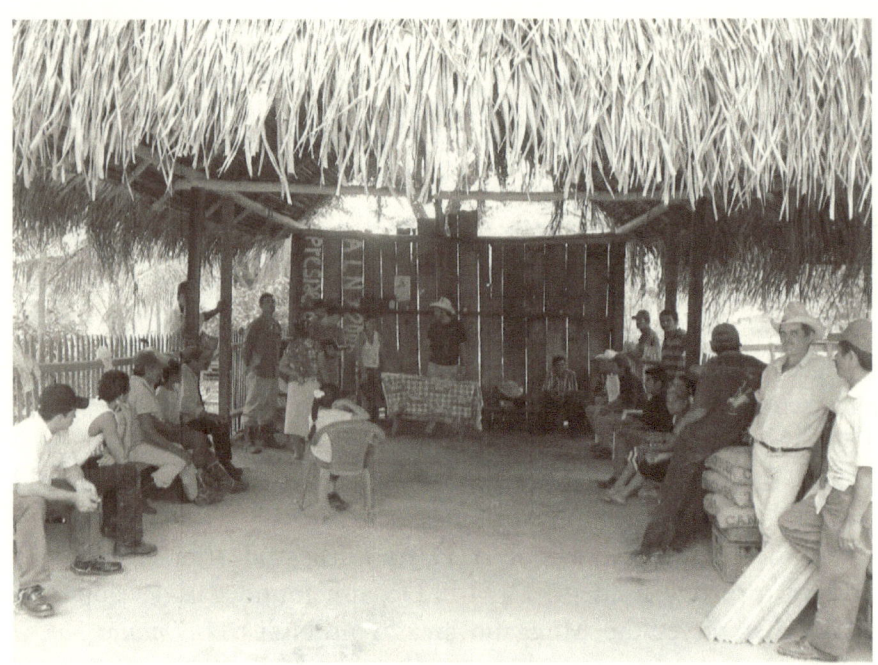

Community training session run by Community Health Workers trained by
Hermanos Por La Salud (www.hermanosporlasalud.org).

Expansion and Barriers: Lawrence Family Medicine Residency would like to expand its global health programming. It is restricted by the Residency Review Committee requirements, which do not explicitly credit global health experience and have extensive requirements spanning the 3 years of residency. Allowing residents to take 4 years to complete residency would permit completion of more global health activities.

Contact information:

Scott Early MD
SEARLY@glfhc.org

University of California, San Francisco Global Health Clinical Scholars Program

Year Established: 2006

Location: San Francisco, California

Discipline: Multi-residency as well as nursing and dental school participation

Website:www.globalhealthsciences.ucsf.edu/education/ClinicalScholars/

Distinguishing Features

- Multi-residency plus nurse and dental school participation
- 3 weeks full time (6 hour/day) course
- Opportunity for a one year competitive program fellowship after training
- Commitment and affiliation with local global health-related organizations
- Mentored scholarly projects
- Meetings bimonthly throughout the year
- International/immersion experiences of varying length (average 2 months)
- Program is an addition to participant's current training

Participation: 24 scholars from seven residency programs and nursing and dental schools. They were chosen from more than 400 possible applicants.

Established field sites: Kisumu, Kenya. Kampala, Uganda. Muhimbili, Tanzania.

Funding: Funding is provided by UCSF Global Health Sciences (GHS) for a faculty director to operate the program (0.2 FTE) with administrative support. Private donors fund a one-year fellowship and support five projects for participants.

Faculty support: 25 core faculty; 100 hours dedicated to global health issues in course, plus 50 hours in evening sessions.

Time residents spend abroad: Varies from 4 weeks to 6 months

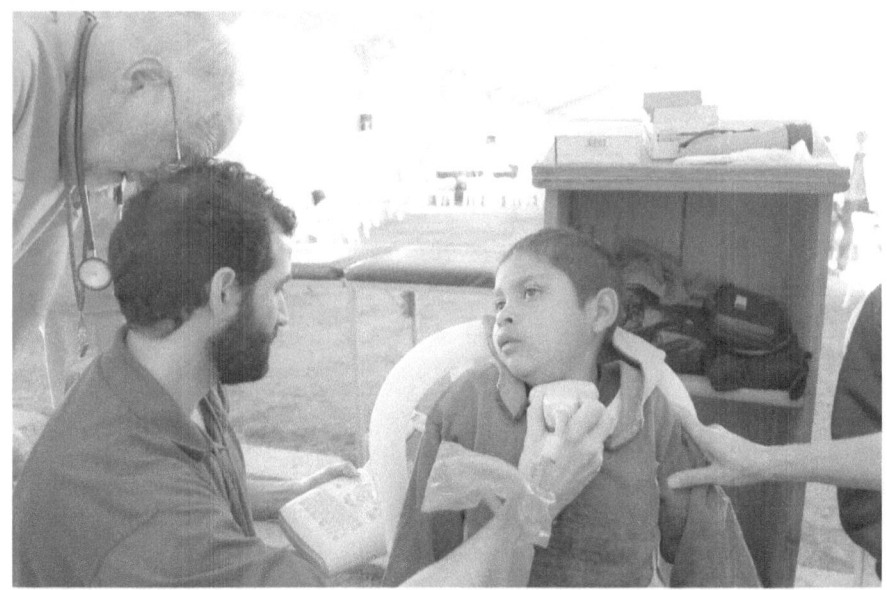

Photo by Terry Burns

UCSF Surgical Resident and Global Health Clinical Scholar Ramin Jamshidi, MD ultrasounds a patient in Botadero, Guatemala.

Curriculum structure: The curriculum includes structured course work during 3-week full-time course; a required project to be completed over 1-3 years of training; evening conferences for journal reviews, invited speakers, documentary viewings, or project reviews; field service with a local immigrant clinic and outreach program.

Description:

This program in global health is unique in that it crosses disciplines. It began in 2006 and is still developing curriculum. It mixes residents from diverse specialties like surgery and psychiatry, coming together with the common interest in global health as a desired part of a career path. Now in its second year, the program has expanded to include equivalent level participants from the nursing and dental schools at UCSF.

The goals of the program are to:
- Develop a cohort of scholars with similar interests in different specialties.

- Teach basic global health principles through a range of fundamental topics.

- Increase networking opportunities with global health faculty.

90

•Provide exposure to multiple career paths within global health.

•Foster interdisciplinary scholarly work in global health within UCSF clinical training programs.

•Encourage commitment to global health issues at home

http://www.globalhealthsciences.ucsf.edu/education/ClinicalScholars/Goals.aspx

The range of topics in global health is so broad that the program does not to try to teach tropical diseases in depth, but rather to develop vocabulary and some skills for global health work. The program is centered on a 3-week full-time course that attempts to explore areas that are not specific to any one discipline, like economics, politics, ethnography, and ethics. Issues such as work-force shortages are examined, and participants work on problems in small groups to better understand them. Although some basic topics are examined in-depth, the course is intended to provide an overview of important global health issues, the vocabulary used in various disciplines, and suggest resources for further study. Another focus of the course is to expose participants to paths leading to a global health career, not just to conduct research or visit a country occasionally throughout a career. Other options are presented through guest speakers or session leaders. Participants organize evening sessions every other week throughout the year.

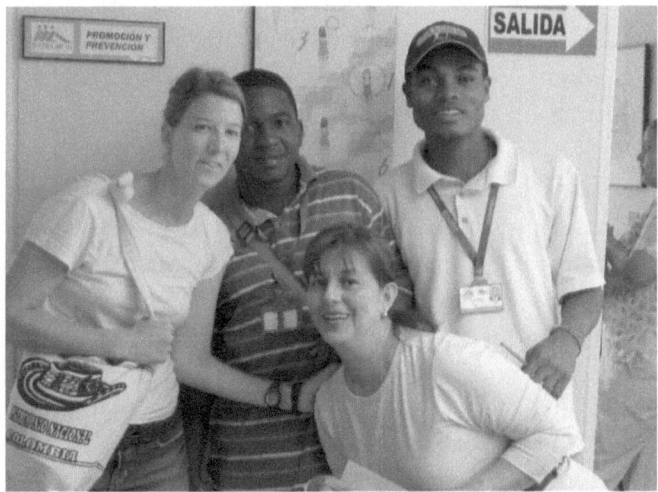

UCSF Master's in Nursing student and Global Health Clinical Scholar Nora Sheedy (far left) with members of a multidisciplinary home visit team in Cali, Columbia.

Projects are done by individual residents, although there is an emerging focus on group projects. Examples of projects are posted on the website. Mentors are available from all departments and schools; it is challenging, however, to ensure that they participate and are given incentives to be involved, especially with so many participants. There is an opening for a fellow to start next year to work in an international setting with support from UCSF Global Health Sciences.

The main challenges faced in creating this program include finding adequate funding, scheduling residents and nursing students from a variety of departments and programs, and providing innovative curriculum development. As the program evolves, it will have to ensure good mentorship and adequate time for project work, given busy resident schedules. Since the program is incorporated into existing educational programs, it is difficult to carve out more time than the course and immersion experiences allow for adequate attention to projects. An additional challenge is to continue interactions over time and after the end of the program among the various participants. Attracting support from other departments and schools for a long-range program also requires persistence.

Data are being collected on this program, but since this is only its second year, the evaluation is limited. The results to date have been positive, and many residents are pursuing research in international settings after graduating. There is clearly much enthusiasm for the program, and competition for spots is only likely to increase. Long-term effects and knowledge and skill acquisition remain to be assessed. Some needs identified in formative evaluation include a desire for funding of international travel and better mentorship support for projects.

On-line cases and further case studies will be developed. At present, the course sessions are recorded and available for participants to review. The program would like to produce shared video lectures with slides and is working on using them to show participants how the issues they learn about affect their interactions in the clinical setting. A relationship is being formed with an immigrant clinic at a county hospital to provide a site for involvement of participants in group projects and individual service.

Contact information:

Chris Stewart MD
cstewart@sfghpeds.ucsf.edu

The Mark Stinson Fellowship in Underserved and Global Health, Contra Costa Regional Medical Center-Family Medicine Residency

Year Established: 2006

Location: Martinez, California

Discipline: Family Medicine, 2-year postgraduate fellowship

Website: http://www.cchealth.org/groups/stinsonfellowship

Distinguishing Features

The fluid world of theory and application in underserved/global health care demands some specialization. This fellowship therefore seeks to prepare professionals who are self-starters and not afraid to ask the difficult questions that confront physicians seeking to provide "health for all." As an innovative program outside traditional academic confines, it will offer fellows an opportunity to explore relationships with local and remote communities on a small scale. Current ethical concerns will be a focus of study, encouraging fellows to join in debates and research on brain drain, inequities in underserved populations in the United States, the role of social justice in health care, and program funds that focus only on specific diseases such as HIV/AIDS or malaria.

Participation: One or two fellows; new fellow(s) start on July 1.

Program Outline and Goals

The Mark Stinson Fellowship in Underserved and Global Health was established to provide additional education and training to family physicians committed to the care of the underserved. The core philosophy is that underserved communities, in both the U.S.A. and abroad, share similar characteristics and have significant health care needs that must be addressed in a comprehensive fashion. Family physicians, with their traditional training in family and community medicine, can contribute significantly to improving health care provision in underserved areas. Further clinical and procedural training, both inpatient and outpatient, will be combined with academic/didactic courses during the 2 years of the fellowship. One year of the fellowship will be devoted to courses and field work through the School of Public Health at UC Berkeley.

The first year, starting on July 1, will begin with orientation and early clinical work and integration with residents, faculty, and staff at the Contra Costa Regional Medical Center. While starting to assume a staff physician role, as either a board-eligible or board-certified family physician, the fellow will be expected to act as a junior faculty member. The academic coursework will begin in late August and continue for two full semesters. During this time the fellow will continue to perform approximately 8-12 hours of work in the county, either in clinical or hospital settings. The academic calendar will guide vacation, study, and project time until the end of May.

The second year of the fellowship begins after completion of coursework for the professional MPH degree. During this 12-month period, the fellow will become an integral part of the physician community in the county's health system. He or she will have outpatient clinical responsibilities of 16 hours per week; these will generally be family medicine clinics but may also include clinics in general pediatrics, internal medicine, and women's health care, including prenatal visits. About 12 hours will be allotted for inpatient skill building, which may include time spend on labor and delivery, in the operating room, and in the intensive care units. Because the program promotes the beginning of a professional life devoted to education and training – in addition to superior clinical skills and community health – pursuing activities integrated into the teaching mission of the residency will be encouraged.

The remaining portion of each week during Year Two will be devoted to study, research, and initiation of the required project. During the middle of this year, the fellow will be relieved of clinical or teaching responsibilities for 2 months to pursue research and field work. This period will allow the fellow to review the literature on underserved/global health, primary health care, and current educational efforts. Each fellow is expected to complete a paper suitable for publication in a journal or for a high-quality presentation to either the local medical/health community or a conference audience. The completed course work, research initiated, and contacts made during the MPH component will be put into practice by fellows during the second year, preferably by getting involved in ongoing work in either rural or urban underserved communities in California or projects in international settings. These activities are intended to foster a lifelong balance between clinical medical services and public health/academic/community development. Such a balanced professional life may benefit more individuals and communities than the one-to-one relationship traditionally inherent in the role of physician. The central objective of this fellowship is to produce family physicians equally adept at providing clinical and procedural services in underserved areas and leading or participating in efforts focused on sustainable changes in communities that improve the quality of life for its members.

Funding:
Salary, $66,000; County support for UC Berkeley tuition. Usual benefits offered to residents.

Field Sites: Program director has extensive networking relationships in Indonesia, Africa, Central and South America, the South Pacific, and Europe. Relationships have been formed with Refuge International, Global Health through Education, Training and Service, and THE NETWORK: Through Unity for Health (TUFH).

Faculty Support: Promoted by the Faculty Leadership Group. Many current faculty/staff members have global and underserved health experience.

External Linkages: The CCRMC Family Medicine Residency is a 13-13-13 program, well known throughout the United States for its dedication to family medicine and a broad scope of procedures useful in traditional and underserved family practice settings. There are close ties with UC Berkeley School of Public Health, UC San Francisco School of Medicine, UC Davis School of Medicine and the Global Health Education Consortium (GHEC).

Contact information:
Scott Loeliger, MD, MS
sloeliger@ccfamilymed.com

Chapter 5

Developing Global Health Programs: Hurdles And Opportunities

Kevin Chan, MD, MPH, Assistant Professor, The Hospital for Sick Children and Fellow, Munk Centre for International Studies, University of Toronto

Melanie Rosenberg, MD, Pediatric Hospitalist, Children's National Medical Center

Chris Stewart, MD, MA, Assistant Clinical Professor, Department of Pediatrics, University of California at San Francisco

Thomas Hall, MD, DrPH, Lecturer, Department of Epidemiology and Biostatistics, University of California at San Francisco

Residencies and fellowships are increasingly interested in developing global health programs for residents and fellows. However, they confront many challenges and barriers: ensuring high-quality experiences with good mentoring abroad, finding salary support for residents traveling to other countries, and protecting the residency program against liability risks. The central challenge is to build a high-caliber program without adversely impacting other aspects of the residency. This chapter explores the hurdles and opportunities of developing global health programs and offers suggestions for addressing problems within individual institutions.

Curriculum Development

Curriculum development in an emerging field like global health is a complex task. It requires setting reasonable and achievable goals and objectives, identifying existing resources available to develop programs, finding time to incorporate global health teaching within current residency curricula and work hour requirements, and demonstrating the value of global health teaching. Successful curriculum development must ultimately rest on two cornerstones, a marked increase in knowledge about global health and significant changes in attitudes toward it.

Developing curriculum objectives

Global health program development is hampered by the lack of standardized guidelines for "good curricula". Program directors need to decide if they want to develop their own curricula or adopt and adapt other programs. The Accreditation Council for Graduate Medical Education (ACGME) through the Residency Review Committee requires residency programs to develop competency-based guidelines. These can be useful in defining curriculum objectives across various areas of practice and ensuring that global health curricula meet the same standards as other disciplines. Some examples for medicine and pediatrics can be found at: (www.acponline.org/fcim/index.html) and (www.ambpeds.org/site/education/education_guidelines.htm).

Collaborating with medical education experts in your institution will help jump start the process and ensure high-quality curriculum development. One can also use objectives developed by existing programs, described in other chapters of this guidebook. Some objectives are appropriate regardless of specialty (for example, developing cultural competency), whereas others are specific to one kind of activity (like training local health workers in neonatal resuscitation).

Guidelines exist for global health as a supplementary learning experience. Some examples include pediatrics (via the Ambulatory Pediatric Association), Family Medicine (www.aafp.org/online/en/home/aboutus/specialty/rpsolutions/eduguide.html), and Emergency Medicine (www.acep.org/webportal/membercenter/sections/intnatl)

Ideally, a program or curriculum in global health should include opportunities for learning about health and development issues in developing countries as well as a mentored international experience.

Finding the time and resources within a residency program will not be easy. Below are some suggestions that may be useful, along with obstacles that may be anticipated.

Incorporating a Didactic Curriculum

The demand on residency programs to cover required topics and specialties limits the time for teaching about global health issues. As Chapter 2 indicates, a variety of methods of incorporating global health education into residency training are available. These include:

- **Protected teaching time:** Incorporating global health teaching into protected conference time, including noon-time sessions and Grand Rounds, which are generally well attended. Still, the number of global health lectures will likely be limited. "Institutional buy-in" (see below) is important to win the support of residency administration for the incorporation of global health topics.

- **Evening seminar series:** Lectures, journal clubs, films, book discussions, etc., have been used to supplement residency activities in global health education. Resident work-hour requirements, however, have to be considered: institutions may decide that residents who stay longer hours to attend lectures violate their strict work-hour requirements, especially if these venues are a required part of the residency program. Family responsibilities and call schedules are other barriers to participating in evening sessions.

- **Elective time:** Some institutions use elective rotations lasting from one to several weeks to provide training in global health. To reach the greatest number of participants with a superior course, consider partnering with other disciplines within your institution.

- **Self-study:** Using web-based or computer-based modules (see Chapter 8).

- **Partnering:** If faculty members accompany residents on their international experience, this may be the best time for focused, case-based teaching.

Obviously, more than one strategy may be used to incorporate global health teaching into residency programs. Starting with a needs assessment of residents may help identify the best format to implement your program.

Ensuring Quality, Accountability, and Mentorship in Overseas Rotations

Many program directors ask for guidance in finding appropriate training opportunities for residents. Ensuring that international opportunities are safe, accountable, and adequately supervised is extremely important, not only for the individual resident, but to guarantee the program's legitimacy and sustainability. Program directors, therefore, must carefully consider how these experiences will be provided to residents.

The ideal mentorship system will link residents with faculty who are traveling and working abroad and who can supervise them properly. With this arrangement good mentoring is assured, no extra burden is placed on host country faculty, and the faculty mentor can cushion the culture shock of a first global health experience.

In the absence of faculty working or volunteering abroad, here are some alternatives to consider:

- Develop specific relationships with international sites. This is best done through an institutional partnership; however, a faculty member or resident who has already established a relationship with the site might be able to develop appropriate objectives for a resident rotation and ensure adequate supervision. A longer-term commitment helps build relationships with partners abroad to make sure that there is an investment from both sides.

- Identify partners who provide residents with appropriate supervision and teaching and pay attention to resident evaluations. A local physician or other practitioner can serve as a mentor for a visiting resident, with clear expectations set out ahead of time. The ability to communicate is, of course, essential, and language abilities and phone/internet access must be taken into account. Building and keeping relationships takes time. If possible, invite mentors to visit your home hospital/institution and give them the opportunity to learn about North American educational models and/or receive training in medical education.

- Set up formal evaluation processes. Existing evaluation models for elective rotations at home can be a start, supplemented by further questions specific to the site. Resident experiences should be evaluated by their supervisor and hosts, so it is important to ensure communication between sites.

An excellent way to develop a relationship and add prestige to colleagues abroad is to provide host country faculty with adjunct appointments at the North American university. This arrangement can take considerable resources and institutional commitments, but the payoff can be great. For example, University of Toronto's Office of International Surgery invited an Ethiopian surgeon for a one-year fellowship to learn about medical education and surgery and appointed him an adjunct professor at the University. Within a year of his return, he was named dean of medicine. Providing small honoraria to local faculty is a more modest way to help ease the cost/burden of a resource-poor country's faculty participation and to solidify relationships.

Joining existing international partnerships may make more sense than creating one from the ground up, especially for small residency programs or those based outside large institutions. Many existing programs would like to provide a year-round resident or faculty presence at their international sites. Partnering locally and regionally may be an approach that builds a program's capacity.

Networks are being formed in South Asia, Latin America, and Africa that provide short-term medical education learning opportunities. Helping support international colleagues to acquire better skills to teach may help your residents in the long run. For example, the Essential Surgical Skills program in Ethiopia attracts surgeons and surgical assistants from Kenya and Sudan (www.cnis. ca). Similarly, a network has been established to learn about medical education through a consortium of medical schools in East Africa (Uganda, Kenya, Tanzania, Rwanda, and Malawi).

Doing Research Projects Overseas

Many residents who want to conduct research projects may find the opportunity to do these abroad enticing. They should, however, remember this simple dictum: while research is done "on" a community, it must be "owned" by the community. The purpose of research is not just to enhance your curriculum vitae but to genuinely help your partner and communities abroad. So when a resident asks, "Should I do research overseas?" The response must be, "It depends."

What does it depend on? It depends on the importance to the host community or country of the research question, the length of time available, and the accessibility of suitable mentors. Even in the best of circumstances, completing research is time-consuming, and internationally based research in the context of demanding residency training is particularly difficult to achieve. Thus it is often best to have a resident work with a faculty member already doing research abroad, thereby allowing the resident to "piggy-back" one or more research projects onto an existing research protocol. It may also be possible to do research with faculty from developing countries. Such an arrangement provides the additional benefits of doing research relevant to the host country, developing closer relationships with host country faculty, and perhaps bringing residency-based research expertise and support to the aid of the host country researcher.

A resident with specific research questions in mind will need to plan early because it often takes 2 years to interest a developing country colleague, write the protocols, obtain funding, and gain final project approval. Residents must get Institutional Review Board approval both at home and abroad before conducting any research; this can take considerable time abroad, especially if one is not present in the country. Even simple epidemiological studies surveying households can take a long time. Plan for delays and unforeseen circumstances: even the best plans may fail if a key partner falls ill or communities are not involved from the start. Residents should have proper training and guidance in planning and carrying out their project in an ethical and responsible manner. Co-authorship with local practitioners should be strongly encouraged, if not required. Having a local partner(s) serve as lead author in a national journal while the resident(s) is lead author on a sufficiently different article in an international journal can be a useful way to recognize host country collaborators.

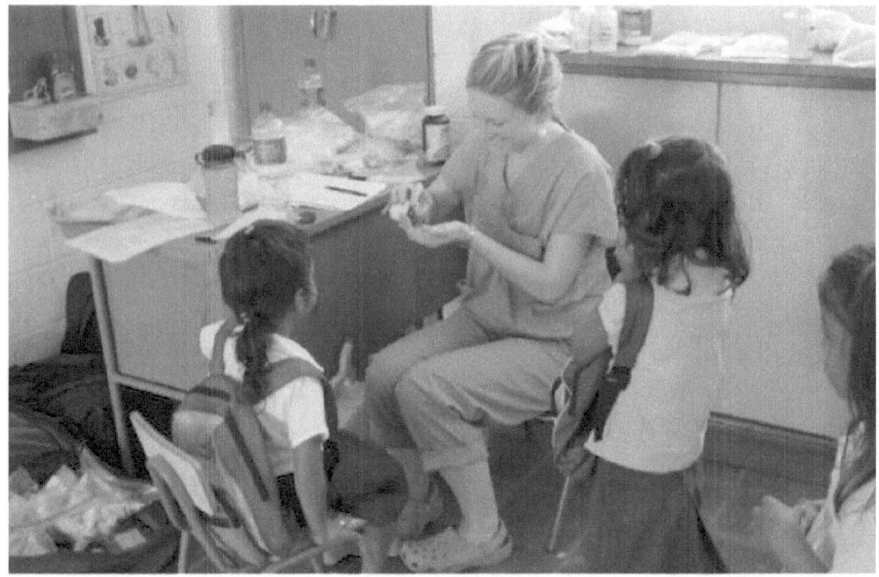

Photo by Kate Nielsen

University of Washington pediatric resident Alison Longnion provides preventive vitamins following country protocols in Abelines, El Salvador with the Children's Health International Medical Project of Seattle (CHIMPS).

Given the short period allowed for most international electives and the time needed to get acclimatized, independent research projects without long-term faculty presence or affiliation will be difficult. Accordingly, most residencies should not require or even encourage overseas research unless they are able to assure adequate preparation and mentorship.

While overseas research may be impracticable, an ongoing service project, without a research focus, may make a good fit with the global health program's goals or requirements, including needs assessments, education or training program development and implementation, assessing equipment needs and maintenance, and setting up new clinics. These activities can meet the expressed needs of local communities in ways that strict research may not, and can be carried out by more than one resident over time. Collecting data and evaluating such projects can provide research opportunities from an evaluation perspective. The same principles of local ownership, involvement, and co-authorship should apply.

Evaluating Global Health Programs

Global health programs should be periodically evaluated for their effectiveness. Evaluation measures should be built into the program from the start and refined with the acquisition of experience. These measures will include monitoring changes in knowledge, medical and/or surgical skills, attitudes toward service, ability to communicate, and career plans. The evaluation framework should take into account changes due both to experiences at the home base and overseas. Demonstrating efficacy and a positive impact on resident education are important to sustain institutional support and funding.

Possible mechanisms for evaluation include the following:

- •Needs assessments of residents before and after implementing a program to determine if it has met their needs.

- •Pre- and post-residency self-assessment by residents, based on curriculum objectives, to determine if the program has met the resident's stated objectives.

- •Pre- and post-assessment of residents by faculty mentors.

- •Pre- and post-tests to demonstrate gains in knowledge base of global health, either before or after a course, or at the start and finish of a residency program.

- •Critical evaluation by residents of all components of the program.

Institutional Support

Support of the hospital and residency program is essential to the development and growth of a global health program. It can take many forms: philosophical, personnel and financial.

Gaining "institutional buy-in" is important from the start. This means convincing hospital and residency program administrators that despite the barriers, global health education is of great benefit, both to individual residents and to the residency program and the international site(s). In developing a proposal for a program, consider the following factors:

- The evidence that global health education has a positive impact on the education and careers of medical students and residents, stimulating interest in both academic programs and serving underserved and immigrant communities (Chapter 1)

- Influence of global health opportunities on choice of residency program. For example, Miller et al.[1] showed that 42% of applicants to Duke University's Internal Medicine Residency considered its global health programs an important factor in their selection. Dey et al.[2] found that 68% of respondents in emergency residencies ranked programs with international opportunities. Federico et al.[3] noted that 67% of the incoming intern class felt that international opportunities were important in the ranking process. Bazemore et al.[4] examined a residency track program and found that the factor most strongly influencing their choice of residency was the international health track.

- Surveying applicants or residents at your institution. An important selling point is that providing global health education may make the residency program more desirable and competitive.

- A needs assessment to demonstrate interest in global health.

- Finding how a global health program fits into an institution's mission. Many centers strive for excellence in both local and international care.

- Providing global health education and help to international sites enhances the public image of hospitals.

- Contribution of the program to academic pursuits, such as writing and research, are important at some institutions.

Accreditation Council for Graduate Medical Education (ACGME) Requirements

Another obstacle to providing resident experiences abroad lies in the Accreditation Council for Graduate Medical Education requirements for residents in a particular specialty. The Resident Review Committee (RRC) for many specialties sets patient numbers and consecutive week quotas in clinics to ensure continuity. Residents traveling abroad often cannot provide continuous care. Since this requirement is tied to funding from Medicare, one solution may be to fund resident slots independent of Medicare and to seek RRC exemption for global health pathways.

A related obstacle is the limited elective time available during a residency. Taking 1-2 months out of residency could be seen to detract from learning the basic competencies and limit the number of resident procedures required to define "competency", especially in surgical programs.

Minimizing Liability Risks

Many residency programs struggle to protect against liability risks arising from residents and their families traveling abroad and litigation from patients in other countries. Residents may have to care for severely ill patients in situations where laboratory tests, x-rays, staff, and consultant support are inadequate. Some bad outcomes are unavoidable. Up to now, liability cases have been few and injury damage awards small – a situation that will probably change as more residents travel abroad for global health purposes.

Each program needs to develop policies and procedures and make administrative support available to the residents/fellows abroad, in conjunction with a legal department that oversees the residency program. Such policies need to have a clear line of command in cases of conflict or confusion arising among the parties.

Each program should provide pre-travel orientation for residents. It should include information and advice on expected and unacceptable participant behavior, personal health issues (including travel advice and immunizations from a Travel Clinic), contingency advice in case problems arise, and the availability of support in cases of adverse outcomes. In addition, it should emphasize the importance of not providing services beyond their current level of competence – an admonition that may be hard to honor when confronted with very sick patients in a low-resource situation.

Residents should be advised that if they do not follow guidelines they will be warned and may be removed from the project site. A faculty member or overseas site mentor should be given the authority to remove a resident.

Communication is also important. E-mail and mobile phones should be used whenever possible, and if good on-site mentoring is not available, the resident should send brief progress reports to his/her home-base mentor at agreed-upon intervals.

Residents who participate in global health rotations need to sign a waiver, acknowledging the risks of working and traveling abroad. They should also provide a one-page information sheet containing next of kin, travel plans, passport and visa information, and affirm that they have reviewed country information from the U.S.A. State Department web site (or the Department of Foreign Affairs and International Trade in Canada). This information should be stored either in the residency program administration or the global health center and form part of the orientation. As part of the consent, each resident should confirm having made provision for travel, health, and evacuation insurance. One good source of insurance is International SOS Insurance (www.internationalsos.com), but a number of other reputable companies are available. As a suggested guide, a minimum of $100,000 medical insurance coverage plus travel evacuation insurance should be provided.

The following pre-rotation guides may prove useful:

- Global Health Education Consortium (GHEC). The GHEC Guidebook: Advising Medical Students and Residents for International Health Experiences. (http://www.globalhealth-ec.org/GHEC/Resources/IHMECguidebk_resources.htm)

- Paul Drain, Steve Huffman, Sara Pirtle and Kevin Chan. Caring for the World. Toronto: University of Toronto Press (to be published in 2008).

- Module 93 of the GHEC module project. (http://www.globalhealth-ec.org/GHEC/Home/Modules.htm)

Impacts of Overseas Placements on Other Residents

Global health residency programs may find that residents not involved in the global health track are increasingly resentful of those who travel abroad, leaving them with heavier workloads and more frequent on-call schedules. Program directors will need to ensure that the on-call burden is equally divided among all residents throughout the year. Following are possible solutions:

- Residents are given "call-free" electives in which they travel abroad.
- Residents should "make-up" their call.
- Continuity clinics: Policies should be established and be flexible so that residents can meet clinic requirements, making up days and still do an international elective.

It is important to create an environment in which schedule changes are supported by administration, faculty, and residents. Interaction between home-based and traveling residents can enhance the residency learning experience by requiring global health residents to share what they've learned abroad with other residents and faculty by presenting at conferences or other venues.

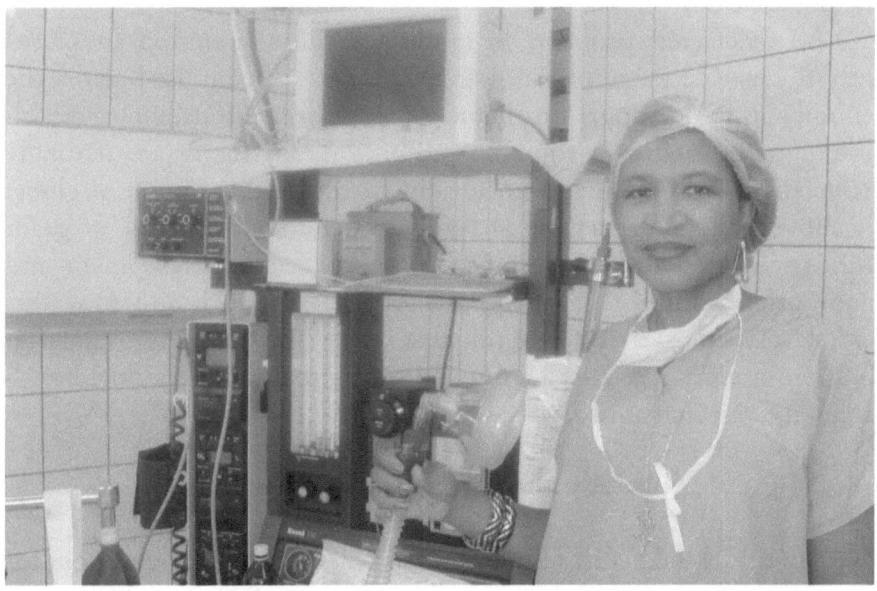

University of Pittsburgh Global Health Program in Reproductive Sciences partners in Swaziland, donating equipment and related training.

Obtaining Salary Support

A chief concern of residency program directors is obtaining funding to support resident salaries while abroad. Salary support is often tied to on-site services at home hospitals, and when residents/fellows travel abroad, the resulting shortfall in revenue leads to reluctance to support global health activities. Many programs seek and obtain independent support for resident international electives, either by using discretionary departmental funds or by appealing to outside donors (individuals, medical alumni funds, or foundations). Some alumni classes have created a program by setting up an endowment for a "global health residency position." One of the best established relationships is between the Johnson and Johnson Foundation and Yale University. The program, known as the Physician Scholars in International Health, supports many residents going abroad (http://info.med.yale.edu/ischolar/). The Hubert Foundation has provided $5 million to Emory University to develop a global health in residency and public health initiatives. A more recent example is a grant by the Bill and Melinda Gates Foundation to the University of Washington; it is allowing the development of opportunities for residency programs in global health.

An associated problem is funding faculty interested in global health. A wide range of funding approaches is being used across the country to find support for them. At most institutions, global health is not recognized as a route to promotion, so faculty are naturally reluctant to become involved. Ideally, to ensure the growth of global health expertise, departmental funds, general endowments, or grant funds will need to be invested to support faculty development and appropriate administrative support. As more global health programs are developed, clear criteria must be established for the evaluation and promotion of faculty who spend substantial time in global health teaching, research, and service.

Family and Overseas Experiences

"Should I take my family abroad?" is a common question for residents planning to spend more than a few weeks away. Any family member who accompanies the resident while traveling should follow the same guidelines and requirements as the resident, as improper behavior could damage the resident's opportunities. Similarly, family traveling abroad should accompany the resident for training and orientation, as they need to be aware of security, health, and welfare issues. Family members will need to make similar preparations regarding logistics, vaccinations, visas, and passports. Residents who decide not to travel with the family will need to consider the implications for those who remain behind. This includes travel duration and expectations, communication arrangements, and support.

Living and working abroad has many life-enriching benefits. Even if your time away is limited, it can help you become a better doctor in whatever field you choose. However, there are career risks to keep in mind. For potential North-American-based employers, will the time abroad be a plus or a minus? Sadly, unless the position is chosen wisely, it could prove a hindrance. Some jobs in North America will give credit towards career advancement for overseas experience, especially in some government, academic, and consultant organizations. For others, however, on return to North America they may find that many colleagues have advanced farther. This may not be a serious consideration for those with a strong commitment to global health, especially those wishing to have a lifetime global health career. If, however, you want just a few years of global health work, and if you want to reach the highest level in your chosen career, think about the effect of spending time away from North America. Will this absence enhance or hurt your reputation and chances for advancement? Can you compensate for your absence through professional publications or periodic returns to North America? Would the global health experience more than compensate for a slower pace of advancement in your primary career? Would it be better to do your global health work early, before your career is well established, and then return, or would it be preferable to become well established and then, after your children have left home, go overseas?

All these caveats aside, one of the most rewarding opportunities is to travel and learn with your spouse and children about other cultures, societies, and other world-views. There's nothing like traveling abroad!

Obtaining Other, Non-salary Support

There are other costs to consider when setting up global health programs abroad: travel costs, including plane tickets and in-country travel, visas, passports, travel insurance, and vaccinations. These costs can be substantial, especially in sub-Saharan Africa and South Asia. The two most common sources of funding for residents families are churches or other religious organizations. As a final challenge, in the spirit of equality, programs might consider targeting travel funding support for international electives to residents with fewer resources so that global health experiences are not limited to the more affluent.

A number of institutions seek support from outside donors (such as medical alumni funds or foundations). Some competitive fellowships can also help support travel abroad. These include the following:

- Yale Johnson and Johnson Physician Scholars in International Health: provides a travel award ranging for $1,000-$5,000 (http://info.med.yale.edu/ischolar/description.html)

- MAP International Medical Fellowship: provides 100% of approved round trip airfare to one destination (must spend a minimum of 6 weeks) (www.map.org/site/PageServer?pagename=what_Medical_Fellowship)

- Rotary Foundation Ambassadorial Scholarship (www.rotary.org/foundation/educational/amb_scho?prospect/index.html)

- American Medical Women's Association Overseas Assistance Grant (up to $1500) (www.amwa-doc.org/index.cfm?objectid=2D58A6B9-D567-0B25-54B67C0C9B20E2B5)

- Christian Medical and Dental Association Johnson Short-Term Mission Scholarship (http://www.cmda.org/AM/Template.cfm?Section=Johnson_Short_term_Missions_Scholarship)

- Sara's Wish Scholarship Fund: For young women, pursuing the ideals of bettering the world (ranging from $1,000-$1,500) (www.saraswish.org)

- American Academy of Pediatrics International Child Health Travel Grant ($500)

- Canadian Paediatric Society International Child Health Grant ($750 Can)

Acknowledgements

The authors kindly thank Elizabeth Hillman for her comments and criticisms. As always, any mistakes are solely our own.

References

1. Miller WC, Corey GR, Lallinger GJ, Durak DT. "International Health and Internal Medicine Residency Training: The Duke University Experience." *The American Journal of Medicine.* September 1995; 99: 291-297.

2. Dey CC, Grabowksi JG, Gebreyes K, Hsu E, VanRooyen MJ. "Influence of International Emergency Medicine Opportunities on Residency Program Selection." *Academic Emergency Medicine.* July 2002; 9 (7): 679-683.

3. Federico SG, Zachar PA, Oravec CM, Mandler T, Goldson E, Brown J. "A Successful International Child Health Elective: The University of Colorado Department of Pediatrics' Experience." *Archives of Pediatrics and Adolescent Medicine.* 2006; 160: 191-196.

4. Bazemore AW, Henein M, Goldenhar LM, Szaflarski M, Lindsell CJ, Diller P. "The Effect of Offering International Health Training Opportunities on Family Medicine Residency Recruiting." *Family Medicine.* 2007; 39 (4): 255-260.

Chapter 6

Preparing Residents For Careers In Global Health

Providing mentoring and other guidance for residents with global health aspirations is a critical part of programming. The role of faculty "champions" in both creating and maintaining global health programming should not be overlooked. Some consider that such programming's main goal is to channel pre-residency interest and activities in global health into a career that includes international contributions. Where faculty champions are scarce, networks of global health educators, such as the Global Health Education Consortium, can offer guidance to trainees and residency programs. In addition, local non-profit organizations with a global reach can often supply mentors. It is helpful to provide residents with role models who have enjoyed successful careers in global health. Because these careers have many forms, pathways, and destinations, making aspiring global health activists aware of this rich variety is critical. The potential goals of global health mentoring are numerous and include the following:

- Imparting the skills to make informed decisions in the choice of global health projects, such as evaluation of ethics, community involvement, beneficiaries of international efforts, and potential pitfalls.

- Assisting with a plan to weave residents' global health interests and abilities into their professional careers, taking into account the constraints imposed by financial considerations, time, geography, language, culture, skill set, and other aspects.

●Providing a model for balancing international and domestic demands.

●Serving as an informational reservoir for global health facts/topics/case studies.

●Preparing residents before departure for an international project involving health, safety, geopolitical, and cultural issues.

●Facilitating networking opportunities among residents and accomplished professionals who share their interests.

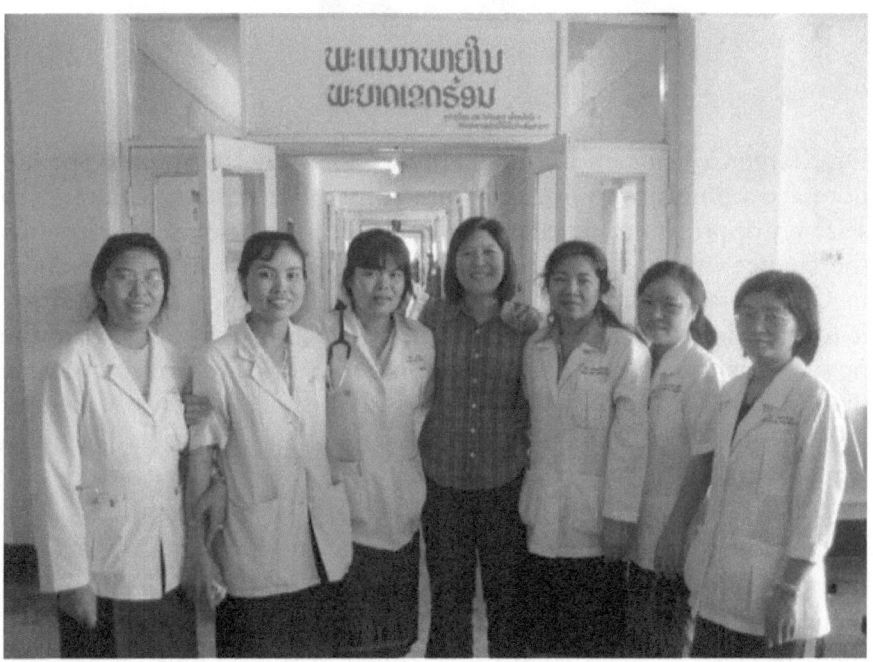

Cindy Chu MD (center red shirt), former Rainbow Babies and Children's Hospital Pediatric Residency International Health Track, pictured here with Laoian residents, is the program's field director in Laos.

Two worthwhile resources are *The GHEC Guidebook: Advising Medical Students and Residents for International Health Experiences* (available at: http://www.globalhealth-ec.org/GHEC/Resources/IHMECguidebk_resources.htm) and *Finding Work in Global Health* (available at: http://www.globalhealth.org/view_top.php3?id=540).

Profiles of Western physicians pursuing global health careers follow. These illustrate the breadth of potential global health careers.

MARGE COHEN

Laura Warner, Medical Student, Rush Medical College

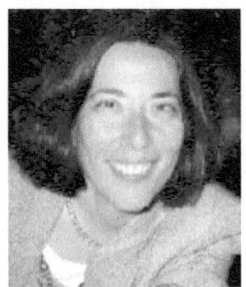

Dr. Marge Cohen came to global health relatively late in life. She did not have aspirations to live and work abroad but was astute enough to seize an opportunity to enter the community of global health when the chance came. Since she had worked with HIV-positive women in Chicago as a clinician and researcher for 20 years, it is surprising it took so long for her to combat HIV/AIDS in Africa -- a role she now sees as a "natural continuation" of her work.. Once she became involved with a group called Women's Equity in Access to Care and Treatment (WE-ACTx), she admits being "bit by the bug" of global health work.

About 4 years ago, Dr. Cohen heard of the need for HIV medications for the women of Rwanda, many of whom became infected through rape during the genocide of 1994. Appallingly, many of these women were sick and dying while the men who raped them received anti-retroviral treatment in prison. This dire need for care led to the formation of WE-ACTx and Dr. Cohen's first trip to Rwanda. The purpose was to establish a clinic where these women could receive the treatment they desperately needed. "That first trip, in April 2004, was when I became committed to the issue", says Dr. Cohen. In the years since, she has returned to Rwanda for 3-4 weeks every few months. One of her main roles in the organization is to raise funds in the U.S.A. for the clinic. Her efforts are aimed at raising "grassroots" consciousness about the cause, as she focuses on reaching out to religious groups, friends, and students.

Through the past few years of developing the clinic in Rwanda, Dr. Cohen and her colleagues have learned how vital it is to be in touch with what their patients need. Apart from HIV medications, they need food, education for their children, and economic empowerment for themselves. The Rwandan people are clearly the best equipped to understand the needs of their own community, thus the WE-ATCx clinic is now staffed by locals. Dr. Cohen says that it took a long time to understand the events of the genocide and its impact on the country. The local people have been an incredible asset for those involved with the clinic, as many of the patients have no addresses or telephone numbers and follow-up can be difficult. According to Dr. Cohen, "it is nearly impossible to find anything unless you've been there before". These lapses in infrastructure contribute to the difficulty of many developing countries in providing all that their citizens need. Many problems stem from the historical exploitation of these countries by colonial powers, making it "impossible for the poor countries of Africa to solve these problems on their own."

Being sensitive to the problems facing developing countries is something about which Dr. Cohen feels strongly. She stresses the importance of those of us in the U.S.A. being "global citizens and [of] feeling that it matters to us what is happening in Kigali as well as in the U.S.A.". This sentiment is directed especially at those interested in global health work abroad. Her advice to those who would like to work in a foreign country is to "follow the lead of the people you know there." Students shouldn't go abroad simply to learn skills, but "to learn about how other people live and to grasp other cultures". Building credibility and relationships with local groups was essential to the success of the WE-ACTx clinic, and simply taking the time to become familiar with local customs made the job easier. Dr. Cohen remembers she had to become accustomed to slowing her pace since "no one is in a rush in Rwanda". Despite being relatively new to global health work, Dr. Cohen is thankful for the opportunity to be involved in such fulfilling work. She has found it hard not to let this project become her major focus now that it has "captured her imagination and desires". She adds, "The friends and colleagues I have met make me feel good all the time", even during times when she is tired or overwhelmed by the sheer amount and gravity of what needs to be done. Dr. Cohen feels privileged to be able to get to know the patients in Rwanda and gratifying to have the tools to help them.

"The desire to help," says Dr. Cohen, "must be tied to understanding in order to produce an impact". While keeping in mind the larger global context and working together with partners abroad to make an impact is the essence of global health. Dr. Cohen asserts that "there is enough money worldwide to have a healthy population in developing countries and we have to demand that". If more of us can find her courage and the strength, perhaps we will someday reach that goal.

NILS DAULAIRE

Regina Crawford Windsor, Master's of Public Health Student, University of Alabama at Birmingham

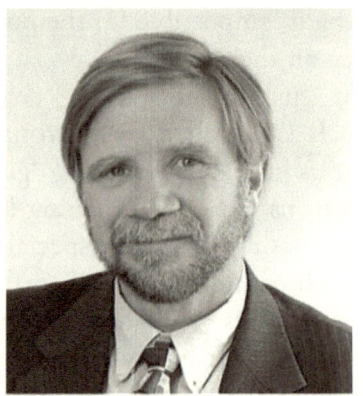

Dr. Nils Daulaire, President and CEO of Global Health Council, began his work in a maternal and child health clinic in Bangladesh. Here he was introduced to the important concept of service to the needy. After initial work with clinicians, he concluded that there were millions of people in need around the globe and that he would never be able to see more than a tiny fraction. He realized that he was more likely to have a lasting impact on global health by affecting the way it is practiced. "Ultimately the importance of how policy was arranged became evident," he asserts.

For 12 years Dr. Daulaire worked as a technical advisor to primary health programs around the world aimed at improving the way programs were conceptualized, how their priorities were identified and formed, and how they were run. What became clear to him was, "you can do a lot with practice and programs, but there are two important mediators." The first is knowledge about what works and how to make the knowledge work for various practical and research programs. The other is realizing that all the knowledge, skills, and methodology in the world are not helpful if the resources and policies that allow people to exercise those skills are not in place.

Dr. Daulaire conducted field research for a number of years on the leading causes of childhood death. Following that, he worked for 5 years in Washington, D.C. as a senior policy advisor at USAID, setting up the framework through which program goals could be accomplished. More recently, as the head of Global Health Council, he has found that effective advocacy groups can have a huge external impact on health policy, "I have a great group of practically-minded practitioners," he comments.

In terms of advice for physicians, medical students, and other health professionals interested in pursuing global health involvement, Dr. Daulaire thinks the foremost objective is to get real-life experience. His time in Washington showed him that there are, "an awful lot of people running around who see themselves as global health experts who wouldn't know the right end of an antibiotic pill . Unless you've actually done it and gone through the challenges of making something work you tend to be very 'ivory tower' and your solutions don't necessarily fit the real world."

The early steps on the global health path are often the most difficult. Dr. Daulaire maintains that there is no specific career path for global health professionals: "There are lots of different ways to get into the field. Having opportunities to work in the field when I was a medical student was probably the critical variable." Those opportunities gave him a chance to be in a clinical setting where he could use his skills and see how to apply them in real-life situations. "After that it was the opportunity of circumstances," he concludes.

In terms of helping future practitioners avoid mistakes, Dr. Daulaire adds, "I think that one assumption is that if you are smart enough, you can figure all of this out without actually having to do it. What I think people need to understand is the complexity of peoples' lives. In poor communities in the developing world, the people are right at the edge of existence." It is a challenge to make significant changes in their behavior because of the complex nature of their existence. He continues, "I think that the simple solution some see is, 'Why don't these people just---' and then fill in the blank. That's probably the most common mistake." For years, Dr. Daulaire and his wife, who works in the field as well, believed that if people would just make sure that their children had access to clean, boiled water and were not exposed to polluted water, they would not have as much diarrheal diseases. When they moved to Nepal, they brought their children who were 1 and 3 years of age. The family spent several weeks in the village. He and his wife, "with at least three advanced degrees between us, and despite the fact that we were not working full-time, could not keep our own children out of polluted water because it is all around." Dr. Daulaire said the "take-home message" is that you have to change both the physical and cultural environment before people can change their behavior to be more health-conscious.

Balancing domestic careers and personal lives with global health activities has been a challenge for the Daulaires. The easiest time was when the whole family lived oversees and they did not have to travel to, "work our trade." The Daulaires spent many years, "doing parental tag teaming; one travels while the other is home, then we'd switch off and that's a real challenge and it drives a lot of people out of the field because it makes it rather difficult for people who are raising families. On the other hand, living oversees with them was a terrific experience."

Dr. Daulaire encourages practitioners to spend time in the field and, "not just in the capital cities and fly-through experiences where you stay in hotels, but actually spend time in rural areas and slums, in settings where people are getting their care." Instead of producing theoretical concepts that do not have a place in their lives, spending time in the field fosters understanding of the realities of peoples' lives. "Respect and understand that there are valid reasons why people behave the way they do, and until you understand and respect that, then you don't get the opportunity to make change," he asserts.

The rewards Dr. Daulaire gets from you global health work are innumerable: "I get to see sometimes, not always, what I consider 'tectonic' changes in the condition of the lives and health of large numbers of people; I feel I've made a contribution to that." From a personal standpoint, the opportunity to see different places, cultures, and societies has been enormously rewarding. He also maintains that one certainly does not go into global health to get rich: "People in the clinical arena who are looking for high income should look elsewhere."

ROBERT GILMAN

Kari Yacisin, Medical Student, Wake Forest University School of Medicine

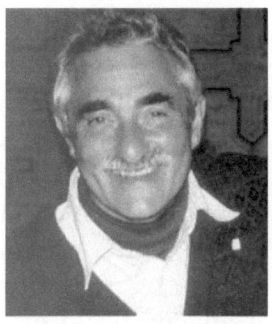

Dr. Bob Gilman's recipe for life goes something like this: mix one month in Maryland with one month in Peru; add several heaping trips throughout South America; a dash of travel to the U.S./Europe; add any other trip, season to taste. Repeat. He commands his career in global health like a master chef, and just as a master chef has had to learn and earn his command, so has this physician-scientist.

Go westward (or eastward...southward...northward...) my friend

Bob Gilman was a kid from New York City who decided to go to medical school. After finishing college in Maine, he did not stray far, attending Downstate Medical College. He acquired a taste for global health when he took a year off after his second year of medical school and went to Europe. After completing medical school and internship, Gilman went westward to an internal medicine residency in Utah.

After 2 years of residency, Gilman applied for an NIH overseas fellowship (no longer in the NIH coffers) and traveled to Malaysia for 3 years to work for the U.S. Navy. There, he fell in love with tropical medicine: "I worked with Aborigines... [it was] fun, exciting... frustrating, hard, but I enjoyed it." Gilman found a satisfying aspect of tropical medicine in that you "feel like you can make an impact." If you are interested in global health, Dr. Gilman emphasizes that living abroad is essential: "Do you want to do it [global health]? Take a year off and see if it fits…You need to spend time overseas." He adds that 1-2 months are not enough, recommending a stay of at least 6 months abroad.

After Malaysia, Dr. Gilman returned to the U.S., completed residency, and identified a program with an overseas global health program (University of Maryland), where he completed a fellowship in Infectious Diseases. Building his career, he went to Johns Hopkins--- first to its Department of Medicine, and, later, to its School of Public Health.

If you have gone abroad and decide to pursue global health as a career, Dr. Gilman recommends being persistent and choosing a site where you feel comfortable, and that has some infrastructure. Do not forget to choose a location for which you will be able to get funding. After all of these considerations, Bob Gilman headed south--way south---of the border: Peru.

Capacity Building

Bob Gilman has spent 18 years in Peru building capacity. "Collaborates" would be an understatement. His group in Lima consists of dozens of individuals—from professors in the local medical school and physician-scientists from the U.K. to local nurses, graduate/college students, and support staff to a perpetual flux of visiting professors and foreign students experiencing life and research in Peru. Their global health efforts revolve around the epidemiology and characterization of various infectious diseases, most recently tuberculosis, malaria, cystercicosis and *Helicobacter pylori*: "The thing we do different is our lack of concentration; research takes on part of your personality."

His lab, which involves laboratory science, behavior intervention programs and field work, strives to focus on "the big diseases that matter in South America," and "to concentrate on things that may have an impact at some point." They want generalizability of their research to other parts of the continent and other parts of the tropics.

Global health efforts are often criticized for being paternalistic and too focused on Western values. With almost two decades in Peru, how has the Gilman Lab addressed this? Dr. Gilman puts it bluntly: "We train Peruvians so that they're smarter than us. We put them in a position where they don't need us." This transition involves the cultivation of paper-writing skills, grant-writing skills, grant-funding, and obtaining positions for individuals in local universities while maintaining their international collaboration. Often, after students in the lab complete medical/veterinary school or earns a Master's at one of the local universities, Bob finds means to train them at Johns Hopkins for 2 years, then has them return to Peru to complete their work. The essential piece, Gilman believes, has been training Peruvians in Peru, having them write their theses in Peru so that their findings are pertinent on a local—if not regional—level. The Gilman Lab essentially follows the mantra of *Think Globally, Act Locally*.

Realities of Money, Medicine and More

Dr. Gilman does not romanticize a career in global health. He repeatedly mentions the financial stress of the job—the endless search for grant money and the risk of losing financial support—and says knowing how to write a good grant proposal is critical. He emphasizes that where "a clinician in the U.S.A. can fall back on skills," if you are doing research abroad, you will need funding and do not necessarily have that financial safety net. Looking back, he wishes he had a stronger background in biostatistics and had pursued an MPH to give him a better theoretical background.

Even with the financial risk involved in a global health career and the challenges of science, Dr. Gilman does not lament leaving the clinical realm of U.S. medicine. He calls the U.S. health care system "dysfunctional, highly tiered…atrocious," and is quick to cite how a shanty-town area of Lima has a lower infant mortality rate than Harlem. His public health side shines as he says that experiencing medicine abroad has convinced him of the importance and utility of preventive care. Public health has been invaluable around the world, especially in developing countries.

When the opportunity to move to Lima arose, his wife eagerly agreed, and they moved their family. He is proud to have daughters who grew up in the tropics. The Gilman family eventually returned to the U.S., with Dr. Gilman "commuting:" 2 weeks in Maryland, then 3 weeks in Peru. Over a year ago, he altered his commute to every other month. Even though the perpetual traveling can be tiresome, Bob Gilman loves his work— the achievement, the intellectual stimulation, and "doing something fun" with people he likes. He found a career recipe that has worked for him. And how sweet it is.

Dr. Bob Gilman holds faculty positions at the Johns Hopkins Bloomberg School of Public Health in Baltimore, Maryland, and at the Universidad Peruana Cayetano Heredia in Lima, Peru. His permanent residence is on a farm in Maryland with his wife and many alpaca.

MARTY ROPER

Kari Yacisin, Medical Student, Wake Forest University School of Medicine

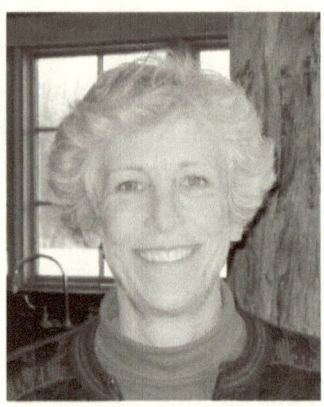

Not all philosophy majors become epidemiologists, but Dr. Marty Roper experienced the transformation, albeit over decades. Originally from Wisconsin, as a young girl Marty dreamed of being a doctor. She went to college, majored in philosophy, and traveled to Germany to work as a lab technician and to study German in order to read Hegel in the original. She realized that she was "not brilliant" in philosophy and that she had "aspirations to do something socially and politically useful." Following her young girl's dream, Marty headed to medical school.

After graduating with a medical degree from NYU, she crossed the continent to begin a residency in internal medicine at Highland Hospital in Oakland, California, and seemed to have settled in to life in the Bay Area. For 15 years, she stayed in Oakland, worked as a supervisor in the Medicine and Emergency departments at Highland, served as medical director of the ambulatory wing of the emergency department, and immersed herself in improving hospital capacity and resident teaching. Dr. Roper became Medical Staff President, and also became antsy. She had achieved much in her career in hospital administration but was eager for fresh challenges. That's when she took a year to travel.

A Traveling Epidemiologist

During this year, Marty volunteered in the south coast swamps of West Papua (Indonesian New Guinea). For 4 months, she conducted a study of malarial drug resistance, assisted with patient care, and took calls for the local medical missionary. She recalls, "I had a wonderful experience…truly in the middle of nowhere….[with] three beds in a little hut." The challenge of medicine in such a remote area —where one "had to use any and everything, [including] your senses"--enthralled her. Global health had hooked her professional and personal interests.

Going from medical practice and hospital administrative responsibilities in the United States to international public health work seems an imposing career change, but for Marty, it was not too radical. In her training in New York City and in Oakland, she treated many immigrants, and she had had an "*i*nterest in working with people from around the world" for many years.

Two ingredients have been critical in Marty Roper's global health career: "meeting people and luck." After her experience in Indonesia, she returned to California, and, following the advice of a mentor, earned an MPH in Epidemiology at the University of California at Berkeley. She then decided to go to London to attend the diploma course in Tropical Medicine and Hygiene at the London School of Tropical Hygiene and Medicine, where she decided that leishmaniasis was a disease she would like to pursue. Her interest in this tropical disease arose from it being a "forgotten, neglected disease, affecting the poorest of the poor…[with] not a lot of competition; a great place to start." On the advice of London faculty, she contacted a researcher at Harvard who needed a visiting scientist to go to Salvador, Brazil, for an NIH-funded project on the inflammatory response to heat treatment of cutaneous leishmaniasis. Marty went to Brazil, where she met a U.S. Army physician working on the development of a malaria vaccine who needed an epidemiologist in the Peruvian Amazon. Marty went to the Peruvian jungle. She later worked for the World Health Organization as a consultant in the Global Polio Eradication Program, spending a year in Pakistan. After a few consultancies for the Centers for Disease Control (CDC), including one in Kenya, she joined the CDC as staff where, as neonatal tetanus were rampant, she helped develop surveillance guidelines for neonatal tetanus in Nepal and reviewed progress in neonatal tetanus elimination in high-priority countries in South Asia. Last fall, through a friend in the CDC, she had dinner with Bob Gilman, a doctor at the Johns Hopkins School of Public Health, and met David Moore, a physician at Imperial College in London, and is now in Peru working to implement the microscopic observation drug susceptibility assay (MODS) in Lima and other sites.

After surviving a mid-life career change, Marty has thrived, and she offers thoughtful advice. She suggests that those interested in careers in global health identify the types of organizations with which they wish to work: do they want to participate in larger organizations that can have greater, albeit slower impact and present the challenges of working in large bureaucracies, or do they prefer to be more independent and join smaller groups, such as non-governmental organizations? If the latter, Marty recommends investigating their histories: are they connected with other organizations, what is their relationship with the local governments, and what is their track record?

Dr. Roper also acknowledges the often complicated dynamic with working in poor-resource settings. She says, "We can go in with best intentions, really listen to the communities, but what keeps things from falling apart? You [have] got to keep asking."

To ensure that working in developing settings does not burden health systems and efforts, Marty recommends reflecting on "how to help in a way that makes sense," adding that, when first arriving in a new setting, it is "best to assume you know nothing about how things work; [problems [persist for] reasons beyond lack of creativity and know-how; solutions that occur to you may already have been tried."

One final challenge that Marty has faced has been that with living and working in so many countries, she lacks a "real" home. So she recently bought a house in Vermont. Overall, this life as a wandering global epidemiologist has invigorated Marty Roper; she says, "I've had a lot of fun, have met really extraordinary people around the world, different points of view, [and] satisfactions from being useful; what I've done is consistent with who I am." Sounds like a true philosopher.

SONAL SINGH

Kari Yacisin, Medical Student, Wake Forest University School of
Medicine

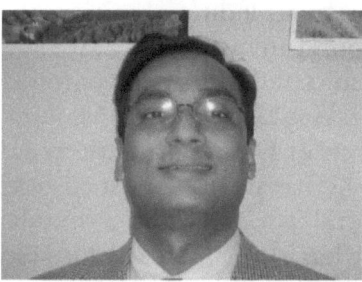

Dr. Sonal Singh misses the mountains. Living in Winston-Salem,
North Carolina, the Blue Ridge Mountains are close, but they are not
the Himalayas of his homeland. Originally from Nepal, Dr. Singh
attended medical school in northern India, and after graduation he
returned to Nepal and worked as a doctor. It was the late 1990s, and
Nepal was experiencing an insurgency. Dr. Singh began to ask how
conflict affected health and health systems, and his career in global
health had unknowingly begun.

A Tale of Two Continents

Wanting graduate medical training in the United States, Dr. Singh
began research involving clinical trials and pharmacology at Ohio
State. He went to the University of Rochester to complete a residency
in Internal Medicine. He chose Internal Medicine because it gave
him "the base, the foundation and the flexibility" to continue pursuing
global health. As a resident, he returned to Nepal during vacations
and met with health professionals, witnessed the situation, and did his
work. He would later join the faculty at the Wake Forest University
School of Medicine in North Carolina.

Caring for the Vulnerable

His research has centered on addressing the health issues of vulnerable
populations (whether in Nepal, North Carolina, or elsewhere), and
the connections between conflict, health, and human rights. Dr.
Singh believes that "society should be defined by how it takes care of
the most vulnerable." He collaborates with doctors involved in non-

governmental organizations and with medical students. (He is currently helping students from London develop a sustainable health program in Nepal, and colleagues from Canada do HIV work in Nepal.) Dr. Singh chose academic medicine because of the credibility it offers. He enjoys working as an attending physician at a medical school and seeing patients. He found an institution that allowed him flexibility for additional career pursuits: he is currently enrolled in a part-time MPH program at the Johns Hopkins School of Public Health. One of the most interesting aspects of Dr. Singh's path in academic medicine and global health is that he has not yet pursued outside funding sources. Not only did his clinical work give him a foundation to address issues in health care, but it has also supported his research time (both as a resident and as a faculty member).

Find Your Passion

Dr. Singh recommends that one interested in pursuing global health "find something you are passionate about," and, "find colleagues also interested" in that passion. He also suggests that young faculty and students understand their roles when working abroad (often limited to pilot projects) and emphasizes sustainability and social determinants: "There is a tendency to look at extremes, but there is a lot more sustainability [locally]; find local things that work rather than de novo." He asks, "How will this work affect people…think about the person…does this writing mean anything to the individual?" Dr. Singh advises not to get discouraged with global health work. A study may not unfold as planned, but keep working. Health issues may become political, but keep working (Dr. Singh even says that one "can be passionately neutral" when health and politics mix.) Time management will often be a challenge, too, but, again, he advises, "keep working."

Thus, although Dr. Singh's career in global health spans two continents, it is united by an emphasis on caring for the vulnerable. His career involves both clinical and research work. His life and career have been multicultural. From Nepal to India to the U.S., Dr. Singh has kept working, and his passion for the health of vulnerable populations led him to a career in global health that holds mountains of possibilities.

Chapter 7

Professional Organizations And Global Health Curriculum: Suggested Guidelines For Pediatric Global Health Training

AAP Section on International Child Health Resident Education
Working Group

Many medical specialty professional organizations have sub-committees that focus on global health. Below is an example of how such organizations can attempt to establish discipline-specific global health curricular standards for resident education. We provide this illustration so that other professional organizations may consider the utility and breadth of such efforts.

These competency-based goals and objectives have been developed by the American Academy of Pediatrics Section on International Child Health working group on Pediatric Resident Education. This group was established in 2006 to address identified barriers to resident education in international health more systematically. These curriculum guidelines were developed in response to the lack of standardized guidelines for international health training in pediatric residencies. They represent a consensus by pediatricians who participate in global health education in numerous pediatric residency programs throughout the United States and Canada.*

These curriculum objectives are intended as comprehensive guidelines for pediatric residency programs offering organized training in global or international health, which might include a didactic curriculum, international experience, or both. They are *not* meant to be prescriptive or encourage requirements for residency programs.

Residency program directors and faculty are encouraged to review these them and adapt them to the needs of individual programs. Residents are encouraged to use and adapt these guidelines to assess their progress in meeting these objectives throughout residency training.

* The objectives were designed using curriculum building tools made available on the Ambulatory Pediatric Association website (www.ambpeds.org) and are based on ACGME competency domains. This website provides curricular material which can be downloaded and customized to each individual program. This document was created using the document "Pediatric Competencies in Brief: Customizable Pediatric Competencies in Brief" found in the Curriculum Building Tools section of the website (registration is required to access this page). The document, which presents the fundamentals of the ACGME competency domains, was then adapted to include competency-based curriculum objectives for international health education of pediatric residents. A more concise set of suggested curriculum objectives for international health are also published on this website under "Supplemental Learning Experiences". As of the time of this publication, the guidelines published here have not been endorsed or published by any professional organization other than the AAP Section on International Child Health.

Source: Kittredge, D., Baldwin, C. D., Bar-on, M. E., Beach, P. S., Trimm, R. F. (Eds.). (2004). APA Educational Guidelines for Pediatric Residency. Ambulatory Pediatric Association Website. Available online: www.ambpeds.org/egweb. [Accessed 02/22/2007]. Project to develop this website was funded by the Josiah Macy, Jr. Foundation 2002-2005.

Primary Goals

GOAL: International Child Health. Understand general principles related to health of children in developing countries and how these principles apply to underserved populations in the United States.

PEDIATRIC COMPETENCIES

Competency 1: Patient Care

Provide family-centered patient care that is development- and age-appropriate, compassionate, and effective for the treatment of health problems and the promotion of health.

1. Use a logical and **appropriate clinical approach** to the care of patients in a developing country setting, utilizing **locally available resources**, and applying principles of **evidence-based decision-making** and problem-solving.

2. Understand the approach to pediatric patients with the following presentations in developing countries and initiate appropriate work-up and management:
   a. Diarrhea/dehydration
   b. Respiratory Distress
   c. Fever
   d. Seizures/Altered Mental Status
   e. Malnutrition (including Severe Acute Malnutrition)
3. Provide **culturally sensitive care and support** to patients and their families.
4. Participate in **health promotion and injury/disease prevention** activities in an international setting, utilizing local guidelines and practices.

Competency 2: Medical Knowledge

Understand the scope of established and evolving biomedical, clinical, epidemiological and social-behavioral knowledge needed by a pediatrician; demonstrate the ability to acquire, critically interpret and apply this knowledge in patient care and community health.

Epidemiology/Public Health:

1. Describe the epidemiology, trends, and major causes of **infant and child mortality and morbidity** in developing countries, and contrast to that in developed countries.
2. Recognize the major underlying **socioeconomic and political determinants** of infant/child health, and how these impact **inequities in child survival** and health care access between and within countries.

3. Describe **known effective interventions, including prevention and treatment**, for reducing under-five mortality and morbidity (e.g., vitamin A supplementation, exclusive breastfeeding, etc.).

4. Describe the epidemiology of **neonatal mortality**, and compare/contrast common causes including perinatal asphyxia and neonatal infections to under-five mortality. Identify **prevention and treatment strategies** (e.g., skilled delivery at birth) specifically aimed at reducing neonatal morbidity and mortality.

5. List the leading causes of **maternal mortality** in the developing world, how they are impacted by health care systems, and contrast them with those in industrialized countries.

6. Identify epidemiological trends and significance of **emerging infectious diseases** in the developing world.

7. Understand the impact of **environmental factors**, including safe water supply, sanitation, indoor air quality, vector control, industrial pollution, climate change and natural disaster on child health in developing countries.

8. Demonstrate a basic understanding of **health indicators** and **epidemiologic tools and methods**, and how they may be used in settings with limited resources to monitor and evaluate the impact of public health interventions.

9. Understand the common childhood **injuries, including drowning, ingestions, burns and motor vehicle accidents** that contribute to childhood morbidity and disability in the developing world, and describe prevention strategies.

Malnutrition and Infectious Diseases:

> 10. Recognize signs and contrasting features of:
> **a. Underweight**
> **b. Stunting (chronic malnutrition)**
> **c. Acute malnutrition – severe/moderate, complicated/ uncomplicated**
> **d. Micronutrient deficiencies (iron, vitamin A, iodine, zinc)**
> **e. Low birth weight** and associated maternal risk factors

Understand and compare the different **anthropometric measures** used to diagnose malnutrition, and principles of **prevention and management** of these different disorders.

11. Describe the interaction between malnutrition/ micronutrient deficiencies and infectious diseases in infants and young children.

12. Become familiar with the presentation, diagnosis, management, and prevention strategies of the following specific diseases in resource-limited settings, based on local and international guidelines:

a. **Malaria** - uncomplicated and complicated/severe (e.g. Cerebral malaria)

b. **Pneumonia**

c. **Diarrhea and dysentery**

d. **Measles**

e. **Neonatal infections** including neonatal tetanus

f. **HIV/AIDS** and related infections/complications

g. **Tuberculosis**

h. **Typhoid Fever**

i. **Dengue Fever**

13. List the **vaccine-preventable diseases** and the immunizations available in developing countries, and know the current international vaccine policies and recommendations (WHO EPI).

14. Identify conditions that contribute to **morbidity and impaired cognitive development** in the developing world such as intestinal parasites, hearing loss, birth complications, anemia, infections (e.g., cerebral malaria), nutritional deficiencies, injuries, and environmental toxin exposures.

Specific Populations:

15. Describe common health issues faced by **immigrant and refugee populations** in developed nations.

16. Describe health issues of children in the developing world affected by humanitarian crisis, including **refugees, internally displaced, and orphans**.

17. Understand the health and psychological impact of certain activities affecting children including **child trafficking, child soldiers and child labor**.

18. Identify specific health issues and needs of **international adoptees**, and describe appropriate screening and counseling for adopting families.

19. Understand the challenges faced by children living with **disabilities** in resource-poor settings, and describe prevention strategies and models of support.

Competency 3: Interpersonal Skills and Communication

Demonstrate interpersonal and communication skills that result in information exchange and partnering with patients, their families, their communities, and professional associates.

1. Appropriately **utilize interpreters and communicate effectively** with families who speak another language.
2. **Communicate effectively and respectfully with physicians and other health professionals** in an international setting, in order to share knowledge and discuss management of patients.
3. Develop **effective strategies for teaching** students, colleagues and other professionals in settings with varying levels of knowledge or understanding of medical English.
4. Demonstrate awareness of **effective communication approaches** for delivery of health care and promotional messages in communities with **limited literacy and education**.

Competency 4: Practice-based Learning and Improvement

Demonstrate knowledge, skills and attitudes needed for continuous self-assessment, using scientific methods and evidence to investigate, evaluate, and improve one's patient care practice.

1. Identify **standardized guidelines** (e.g., WHO/UNICEF) **for diagnosis and treatment** of conditions common to developing countries and adapt them to the individual needs of specific patients.
2. Know and/or access **appropriate medical resources** and apply them to the care of patients in the developing country setting.
3. Understand the **principles of evidence-based medicine** and apply them when reviewing recent literature and considering the implications for impact on practice.
4. **Work collaboratively with health care team members** to assess, coordinate, and improve patient care practices in settings with limited resources.
5. Apply and improve upon **physical examination skills and clinical diagnosis** in settings where diagnostic studies are limited.
6. Establish **individualized learning objectives for an international elective** and strategies for meeting those

objectives.

7. Identify and utilize the **resources needed to prepare for an international rotation** or work in a less developed country.

8. Understand the role of the pediatrician in responding to **humanitarian emergencies and disaster relief efforts**, within the context of participating local and international organizations, and become familiar with available resources to prepare for volunteering in this setting.

Competency 5: Professionalism.

Demonstrate a commitment to carrying out professional responsibilities, adherence to ethical principles and sensitivity to diversity when caring for patients in a developed or developing country setting.

1. Demonstrate a commitment to **professional behavior** in interactions with staff and professional colleagues and be respectful of differences in knowledge level and practices.

2. Give examples of **cultural differences** relevant to care of international populations and how **traditional medicine** and Western/scientific medicine can conflict with or complement one another.

3. Identify **common ethical dilemmas and challenges** confronted when working in a setting with limited resources or different cultural values.

4. Understand the **ethical standards and review processes** for research with human subjects carried out in developing countries.

5. **Recognize personal biases** in caring for patients of diverse populations and different backgrounds and how these biases may affect care and decision-making.

6. **Plan a responsible and ethically-guided international rotation experience**, ensuring adequate preparation and appropriate expectations both for yourself and your international hosts.

7. Understand and be sensitive to the profound **inequities in global health** and how individuals can contribute to diminishing these disparities.

Competency 6: Systems-based Practice

Understand how to practice high-quality health care and advocate for patients within the context of the health care system.

1. Compare and contrast different **health care delivery settings in the developing world**, including hospitals, clinics and the community, and the roles of different health care workers as they apply to patients in developing countries, such as the physician, nurse, community health worker, traditional birth attendant, etc.

2. Identify the **major governmental and non-governmental organizations** active in international child health, and give examples of initiatives and programs that impact child health (WHO, UNICEF, Global Fund, GAVI, etc.). Understand how the policies and funding structures of these organizations as well as donor nations impact global child health.

3. Describe international goals and strategies for improving child and maternal health (such as the **Millennium Development Goals**), and how these have impacted policy, funding and development of newborn, child and maternal health programs worldwide.

4. Develop understanding and awareness of the **health care workforce crisis in the developing world**, the factors that contribute to this, and strategies to address this problem.

5. Identify different **health care systems and fee structures** between and within countries, including the **public and private sectors**, and understand the impact of these systems on access to patient care and quality of care.

6. Demonstrate sensitivity to the **costs of medical care** in countries with limited resources and how these costs impact choice of diagnostic studies and management plans for individual patients.

7. Contrast the advantages and disadvantages of different **approaches to implementing health care interventions** in developing countries, such as vertical or targeted programs vs. integrated; focused vs. comprehensive; facility-based vs. community. Describe the **WHO Integrated Management of Childhood Illness (IMCI)** program as an example.

8. **Advocate** for families, such as recent immigrants to a developed country, who need assistance to deal with system

complexities, such as lack of insurance, multiple appointments, transportation, or language barrier.

9. Understand the pediatrician's role in **advocating for health policy efforts** that can reduce inequities and improve health of children in developing countries.

Please direct any feedback or suggestions on these guidelines to Melanie Rosenberg: mrosenbe@cnmc.org

Chapter 8
Resources For Teaching Global Health

Kevin Chan, MD, MPH, Assistant Professor, The Hospital for
Sick Children and Fellow, Munk Centre for International Studies,
University of Toronto

Chris Stewart, MD, MA, Assistant Clinical Professor, Department of
Pediatrics, University of California at San Francisco

Melanie Rosenberg, MD, Pediatric Hospitalist, Children's National
Medical Center

Thomas Hall, MD, DrPH, Lecturer, Department of Epidemiology
and Biostatistics, University of California at San Francisco

A wide variety of resources are available for teaching global health. The first place to look is within your own hospital and university. You can also find experts from your community and among immigrants from around the world who live near you! However, in the absence of adequate help locally, there are a number of wonderful resources available to teach global health. This chapter highlights some of them.

Global Health Teaching Modules

The Global Health Education Consortium (GHEC) is creating more than 100 peer-reviewed global health modules on various topics in global health. The modules are available on the GHEC website and include PowerPoint slides (in Macromedia "Flash" format) backed up by supplementary notes, case studies, and often, an end-of-module quiz. They can be accessed at www.globalhealthedu.org

(1) *Wellcome Trust:* "Topics in International Health" teaching modules are CDs that can be purchased individually or institutionally. A demonstration of these modules can be accessed at: www.wellcome. ac.uk/node5810.html

(2) *Baylor Pediatric AIDS:* Excellent online HIV curriculum with cases and questions at the end of each chapter (http://bayloraids.org/curriculum/)

(3) *Tufts:* Open CourseWare (http://ocw.tufts.edu/courses/1/CourseHome)

(4) *Swansea with University College Hospital, Ibadan, Nigeria.* (www.medicine.swan.ac.uk/inthealth.html) Five e-Learning modules on: Global Burden of Disease, TB, malaria, HIV/AIDS, Obesity, and an Introduction to Parasitology. They were designed mainly for individual study by medical students at the two collaborating institutions.

(5) *USAID:* (www.globalhealthlearning.org) There are currently 15 modules on global health with an aim to have 48 modules. This website has fun interactive quizzes in each part of the module, with simple presentations.

(6) *University of North Carolina:* (www.sph.unc.edu/general/certificate_programs.html) They have distance certificate programs in the following areas: community preparedness and disaster management, core public health concepts, field epidemiology and public health leadership.

(7) *University of North Carolina, "Nutrition in Medicine" series:*

(www.med.unc.edu/nutr/nim) This is an impressive high-end web-based teaching module with Flash macromedia and includes audio, streaming video, interactive quizzes and drop-down windows.

(8) *Johns Hopkins School of Public Health:* (http://ocw.jhsph.edu) Some of Johns Hopkins School of Public Health's most popular courses are available at the OpenCourseWare (OCW) project.

(9) *The Supercourse: Epidemiology, the Internet and Global Health* (University of Pittsburgh). (www.pitt.edu/~super1) This course is a repository of lectures on public health and prevention, with over 3,000 non-peer-reviewed powerpoint lectures.

Global Health Bibliography

The Global Health Education Consortium has produced a global health bibliography (www.globalhealth-ec.org/GHEC/Resources/GHbiblio_resources.htm), last updated in January 2008. There are 830+ references in more than 25 different categories. A number of good basic textbooks are currently available including: *Understanding Global Health* edited by William Markle, Melanie Fisher and Ray Smego and *International Public Health* (2nd edition) edited by Michael Merson, Robert Black and Anne Mills.

Global Health Websites

The Global Health Education Consortium has produced a recent update in July 2007 of the annotated global health-related websites (www.globalhealth-ec.org/GHEC/Resources/GHonline.htm). Some good places to start include the Centers for Disease Control and Prevention (CDC), the Department of State, the Global Health Council and the Global Health Education Consortium websites (www.globalhealth-ec.org and click on Resources).

Film Documentaries

There are a number of wonderful documentaries and films on global health. Here is a list of some good global health documentaries.
  ¡Salud!. Medical Education Cooperation with Cuba, 2006.

Rx for Survival - A Global Health Challenge. WGBH Educational Foundation and Vulcan Productions, Inc. 2005.
A Closer Walk. Worldwide Documentaries. 2003.
Beyond Borders. Mandalay Pictures. 2003.
Twelve Monkeys. Atlas Entertainment. 1995.

Course Curricula

The Global Health Education Consortium has prepared a guidebook entitled, *"Developing Global Health Curricula: A guidebook for U.S. and Canadian medical schools,"* in collaboration with AMSA, IFMSA and others. Though focused on the needs of undergraduate medical students, parts of this guidebook may have substantial relevance to a residency program. It is available at www.globalhealth-ec.org under "Resources".

Implementing evidence-based medicine in resource-poor settings is an important component of a global health curriculum. The Cochrane Developing Countries Network (http://dcn.cochrane.org/en/localrevs.html) is promoting research, practice, and access to health information and publications for developing countries. Additional teaching EBM resources can be found at http://www.cebm.utoronto.ca/syllabi/devl/.

Training Programs for Faculty and/or Residents

Examples of some of the many training programs that could be relevant for faculty and residents are listed below. Cost, duration, and timing details are as of mid-2007 and are subject to change.

(1) 'The Gorgas Course in Clinical Tropical Medicine' by the Gorgas Memorial Institute and University of Alabama - Birmingham. (http://info.dom.uab.edu/gorgas/index.html) The course includes lectures, case conferences, diagnostic laboratory and daily bedside teaching on a 36-bed tropical medicine unit, is taught in English, and based in Lima, Peru, during 9 weeks from January to March for U.S.A. $5,995 (includes 2 field trips).

(2) 'Program on Ethical Issues in International Health Research' by Harvard School of Public Health. (http://www. hsph.harvard.edu/bioethics) Discusses ethical issues related to

international health work and research. Held in Boston, MA during 5 days in June. Cost is $1,800.

(3) 'The HELP (Health Emergencies in Large Populations) Course' by the International Committees of the Red Cross and Red Crescent Societies (www.jhsph.edu/Refugee/HELP/index. html)   Seeks to upgrade professionalism in humanitarian assistance programmes conducted in emergency situations. Held at Johns Hopkins, Baltimore, MD in July, 3 weeks for $1,500.

(4) 'Summer Institute in Tropical Medicine and Public Health' by Johns Hopkins Bloomberg School of Public Health. (www.jhsph.edu/tropic)   Provides training in tropical medicine and related public health issues in order to prepare participants for working on health problems in developing countries and travelers. Course is four two-week modules. Held in Baltimore, MD during 8 weeks from June to August (participants can take any or all of the two-week modules). Cost: One Module: U.S.A. $1,680; Two modules: U.S.A. $3,150; Three modules: U.S.A. $4,520; Four modules: $5,780 (not including housing).

(5)   'Summer Institute in Reproductive Health and Development' by the Johns Hopkins Bloomberg School of Public Health.   (www.jhsph.edu/GatesInstitute)   Provides training in reproductive health research and enhances leadership skills. The courses address reproductive health and development, combining contemporary issues in reproductive health, research methods and leadership training. The program is designed as two 3-week courses. In Baltimore, MD during 4 weeks in June/July. Cost is U.S.A. $2000 per course. Some scholarships are available.

(6)   'Graduate Summer Institute of Epidemiology and Biostatistics" by the Johns Hopkins Bloomberg School of Public Health. (www.jhsph.edu/summerEpi) Course provides an understanding of basic and advanced principles of epidemiological research, and will present epidemiologic methods and their application to the study of the natural

history and etiology of disease. Held in Baltimore, MD during 4 weeks in June/July. Cost is U.S.A. $2,000 per course.

(7) 'Diploma in Tropical Medicine & Hygiene' by the Liverpool School of Tropical Medicine. (http://www.liv.ac.uk/lstm/learning_teaching/post_grad/DiplTropMedHyg.htm) Course aims to equip physicians with the knowledge and skills needed to practice medicine and promote health in the tropics effectively. Held in Liverpool, UK, during 13 weeks from September to February. Cost is 2,958 British Pounds.

(8) 'Diploma in Tropical Medicine & Hygiene' by the London School of Hygiene & Tropical Medicine. (www.lshtm.ac.uk/prospectus/short/stmh.html) Program combines practical laboratory work, a series of lectures and seminars and some clinical experience and is designed to provide doctors with the clinical and factual knowledge that will form the basis of professional competence in tropical medicine. Held in London, UK, during 3 months from January to March. Cost is 3,850 British Pounds.

(9) 'International Course in Tropical Medicine' by The Louisiana State University Health Science Center & The University of Costa Rica Faculty of Medicine. (http://www.medschool.lsuhsc.edu/student_affairs/electives/MICROBIOLOGY.htm) Course aims to provide students with an insight into the impact of tropical diseases on the population of affected areas. It combines lectures, discussions, laboratory exercises, and some clinical presentations. Students do not participate in direct patient care. Teaching sites include several different region of Costa Rica in July. Cost is U.S.A. $1,500 (not including airfare).

(10) 'Graduate Diploma Programme in Tropical Medicine and Hygiene' by Mahidol University's Bangkok School of Tropical Medicine. (www.tm.mahidol.ac.th/en/academic/bstm/bstm_index.htm) Provides graduates with knowledge of tropical health problems and diseases, including epidemiology, etiology, pathogenesis, pathology, nutritional aspects, risk factors and clinical manifestations. Courses are taught in English and are

held in Bangkok, Thailand, during 6 months from April to September. Cost is US$4,000.

(11) 'International Medicine Course' by Mayan Medical Aid. (http://mayanmedicalaid.org/global_health_ed.htm) Provides participants with immersion, didactic teaching, and the opportunity to practice the information learned in a clinical setting. The course encompasses 10 modules and is held in Santa Cruz La Laguna, Guatemala. Cost is US$710 for first two weeks, then US$320 for each subsequent week. (travel, food, lodging not included).

(12) 'Tropical Disease Biology and Research in Ecuador' by Ohio University College of Osteopathic Medicine. (www. oucom.ohiou.edu/dbms-grijalva) Workshop is held in Ecuador during June and July. Cost is US$1,100-$2,000, plus $150 program fee.

(13) 'Diploma Course in Clinical Tropical Medicine and Travelers' Health' by Tulane University's School of Public Health and Tropical Medicine. (www.sph.tulane.edu/tropmed/ programs/diploma.htm). It provides a structured curriculum with practical instruction in tropical medicine, including the pathophysiology, clinical features, diagnosis, treatment, and control of diseases prevalent in the tropics. Held in New Orleans, Louisiana during 4 months from August to December. Cost is US $10,000. plus US$1,000 for room and board.

(14) 'Course on the Surveillance of Transmissible Diseases' by the UNICEF/UNDP/World Bank/WHO Special Programme for Research and Training in Tropical Diseases and the Swiss Tropical Institute. (www.who.int/tdr/grants/grants/sti_course. htm) The first part of the course will be devoted to general aspects of surveillance of transmissible diseases, illustrated by case studies, and the second part will deal with the functions and importance of the disease notification system. Decision structures and necessary means for the control of epidemics are discussed. Held in Basel, Switzerland during 2 weeks in October/November. Cost is transportation to Basel and stipends are provided.

(15) 'Principles and Practice of Tropical Medicine' by
the Uniformed Services University of the Health Sciences
(http://www.usuhs.mil/pmb/TPH/index.html). It presents
a comprehensive approach to the principles and practice of
tropical medicine. For students interested in qualifying to sit
for the American Society of Tropical medicine and Hygiene's
certifying examination in Tropical Medicine and Traveler's
Health. Held in Bethesda, MD during 13 weeks from February
to May. Cost is US$5,000.

(16) 'International Health in the Developing World' by the
University of Arizona. (www.globalhealth.arizona.edu/IHIndex.
html) A multidisciplinary, case-based, problem-solving course
that prepares medical students and primary care residents
for health care experiences in developing countries. Held in
Tucson, Arizona during 3 weeks in July. Free for medical
students and US$500 for residents and physicians.

(17) 'Global Health Course: Diploma in Clinical Tropical
Medicine and Travelers Health' by the University of Minnesota
Department of Medicine. (http://www.globalhealth.umn.edu/
globalhlth/course.html). Course prepares attendees to work
in global health, including tropical medicine, travelers' health,
refugee and migrant health. Held in Minneapolis, Minnesota
during 8 weeks in July/August.

(18) 'Clinical Tropical Medicine and Parasitology Course' by
West Virginia University. (www.hsc.wvu.edu/som/tropmed)
Course focuses on the essential skills and competencies
required in clinical tropical medicine, laboratory skills in a
low-technology setting, epidemiology and disease control, and
traveler's health, and provided in four 2-week modules. Held
in Morgantown, WV during 8 weeks from June to August.
Cost is US$4,900 for physicians and dentists; $3,800 for
physicians working overseas for charitable NGOs; and $3,400
for nurses, physician assistants, and physicians in residencies or
fellowships.

(19) 'Summer Course on Refugee Issues' by York University's
Centre for Refugee Studies. (www.yorku.ca/crs/summer.
htm) Program offers postgraduate training in refugee issues

for practitioners involved in refugee protection or assistance. It includes panel discussions, case studies, a simulation exercise, and lectures from international experts. Held in Toronto, Canada during 8 days in June. Cost is CAN $850 (does not include food and accommodations).

(20) 'Course on Border Health' by University of Texas (http://steer.uthscsa.edu/course.html)

(21) 'Management of Humanitarian Emergencies: Focus on Children and Families.' By Case Western Reserve University. (http://cme.cwru.edu/course_liveevents.aspx?Course=201) This is an excellent course for anyone planning to do disaster relief. Relatively inexpensive dorm housing is available for residents. Held in Cleveland, OH annually during June. CME credits available.

Interactive Website on Global Health Matters

Among the various interesting interactive websites relevant to global health are the following:

(1) Source. (www.asksource.info/index.htm) The International Information Support Centre seeks to strengthen the management, use and impact of information on health and disability worldwide. Its "Resource Library" contains a wide variety of information including details of books, reports, websites, organizations, newsletters and more. You can browse selected and reviewed resources in key topic areas, or search the full range of subject areas in our three online databases.

(2) GapMinder (www.GapMinder.org). Highlights global gaps in health and poverty.

(3) WorldMapper displays information in maps (www-personal.umich.edu/~mejn/cartograms). World social, economic, health and other indicators are portrayed on global maps that reflect not the size of countries, but the relative size of their GDP, population, energy use, health indicators, etc.

(4)   Population Reference Bureau (PRB) is an excellent source of population-related data relevant to global health (http://www.prb.org/datafinder.aspx). The data bank includes many tables and graphs in downloadable Powerpoint files.

(5)   Global Poverty Mapping Project (www.ciesin.columbia.edu/povmap/index.html)   This atlas provides examples of the important uses of poverty maps, including: the ability to overlay them with maps of geographical features, agro-ecological zones, education, accessibility, services and so on, so as to better understand and analyze possible causes of poverty, for better targeting of resources, and for raising donor awareness of financing needs.

(6)   UNICEF Customized Statistical Tables (www.unicef.org/statistics/index_24183.html). Using data from the most recent State of the World's Children, users can choose indicators and compare by region or country, generate tables exportable to Excel.

(7)   Millennium Development Goal Indicators (http://millenniumindicators.un.org/unsd/mdg/default.aspx)

Conferences

(1) Western Regional International Health Conference sponsored by the University of Washington, University of Arizona, and Oregon Health Sciences University.

Location: Rotating throughout the western United States
Month: February
Website: depts.washington.edu/ihg

(2) Global Health Education Consortium Conference

Location: Rotating in North America and Central America
Month: during February – April period
Website: www.globalhealth-ec.org

(3) Unite for Sight International Health Conference

Location: Rotating in the United States
Month: April
Website: www.uniteforsight.org

(4) The Mount Sinai Global Health Conference

Location: New York City
Month: April
Website: mssm-ghc.org

(5) Northern California International Health Conference sponsored by the Bay Area International Health Interest Group, University of California - Davis, University of California - Berkeley, University of California - San Francisco, Stanford University, and Kaiser Permanente.

Location: Rotating in northern California
Month: March or April
Website:
www.ucdmc.ucdavis.edu/cme/Confrnce/8thAIHC/ConfrncePage.htm

(6) International Conference on Global Health of the Global Health Council

Location: Washington D.C.
Month: May/June
Website: www.globalhealth.org/conference

(7) International AIDS Conference by the International AIDS Society

Location: Rotates globally.
Month: August
Website: www.iasociety.org

(8) International Conference on the Scientific Basis of Health Services

    Location: Rotating globally and held every two years.
    Month: September
    Website: www.icsbhs.org/index_eng/html

(9) WONCA Rural Health Conference

    Location: Rotating around the world.
    Month: September
    Website: ruralwonca2006.org

(10) WIDER (World Institute for Development Economics Research) Conference

    Location: Rotates globally
    Month: September
    Website: www.wider.unu.edu

(11) Canadian Conference on International Health

    Location: Ottawa, Canada
    Month: October/November
    Website: http://www.csih.org/en/ccih/index.asp

(12) American Public Health Association

    Location: Rotating in the United States
    Month: November
    Website: www.apha.org/meetings

(13) American Society for Tropical Medicine and Hygiene

    Location: Rotating in the United States
    Month: November
    Website: www.astmh.org

(14) Global Missions Health Conference by the Southeast Christian Church

Location: Rotating in the United States
Month: November
Website: http://www.medicalmissions.com/conference

www.ingramcontent.com/pod-product-compliance
Lightning Source LLC
Chambersburg PA
CBHW020435290526
45785CB00002B/867